Vulnerability and Care

T & T Clark
Religion and the University Series

Volume 4:
Vulnerability and Care: Christian Reflections on the Philosophy of Medicine

The *Religion and the University* series is concerned with the revitalization of Christian culture through the reform of the university and more widely with the revitalization of religious culture through university education. The series aims to demonstrate a creative and imaginative role for the Christian theological perspective within the university setting. Contributions to this series are welcome, and prospective editors and authors can find further information at http://www.bloomsbury.com/uk/series/religion-and-the-university/

Vulnerability and Care is the fourth volume in the series. Andrew Sloane provides Christian philosophical and theological reflections on the nature and purposes of medicine and its role in a Christian understanding of human society. Medical and bioethical issues have spawned a great deal of debate in both public and academic contexts. Little has been done, however, to engage with the underlying issues of the nature of medicine and its role in human community. This volume brings together a variety of philosophical and theological reflections to emphasize the Christian understanding of medicine as both a scholarly and social practice.

Vulnerability and Care

Christian Reflections on the Philosophy of Medicine

Andrew Sloane

Bloomsbury T&T Clark
An imprint of Bloomsbury Publishing Plc

BLOOMSBURY
LONDON • OXFORD • NEW YORK • NEW DELHI • SYDNEY

Bloomsbury T&T Clark
An imprint of Bloomsbury Publishing Plc

Imprint previously known as T&T Clark

50 Bedford Square
London
WC1B 3DP
UK

1385 Broadway
New York
NY 10018
USA

www.bloomsbury.com

First published 2016

British Library Cataloguing-in-Publication Data
A catalogue record for this book is available from the British Library.

ISBN: HB: 978-0-56731-677-6
ePDF: 978-0-56740-977-5
ePub: 978-0-56700-108-5

Library of Congress Cataloging-in-Publication Data
A catalog record for this book is available from the Library of Congress.

Typeset by RefineCatch Limited, Bungay, Suffolk
Printed and bound in Great Britain

Contents

Acknowledgements

The acknowledgements at the start of a book are an odd beast. An author talks to a bunch of people their readers are unlikely to meet, expressing gratitude for the way those unknown people have contributed to a book that the readers are not yet sure they're particularly thankful to read. They are important, nonetheless: for they don't just thank the people whose names don't appear on the cover for the contribution they make to what's inside it; they also acknowledge that books, even monographs, are not the achievements of an isolated individual, but grow out of rich conversations and creative relationships. They are, in short, the product of communities. The acknowledgements give authors the opportunity to part the curtains of publishing and share the stage with their 'crew'. To step out of the limelight for a moment and bring them out of the shadows to receive their due applause – and to do so before the audience has a reason to boo.

So, I hope you will join me in thanking the following . . .

Morling College, Sydney: to the Board for generous provision of study leave and the funding that allowed Alison and me to travel to London on sabbatical; to colleagues for encouragement and conversation and taking up the slack while I was gone.

St Mary's University, Twickenham, and particularly the staff of the Centre for Bioethics and Emerging Technologies, and the Director of the Masters programme in Bioethics and Medical Law, Dr Trevor Stammers, for welcoming me as visiting scholar. Trevor gave generously of his time and knowledge (and even his office space) to an Aussie bloke he'd never met. Thanks for many chats over coffee and lunch (and the occasional pint). Yes, they helped greatly as I wrestled with tricky questions; but just as importantly, they were a wonderful expression of Christian fellowship and hospitality which made our time in London a richer and happier experience.

Peter Hampson, for the invitation to contribute to this series, and his warm hospitality and engaging conversation in Oxford.

Neil Messer, for stimulating discussion in Winchester. We don't always agree, but he helped me to think better about medicine.

The kind people of Teddington Baptist Church (especially the pastor, Richard Littledale), for giving us a spiritual home during our time in London.

James and Sue Clarke, for a lifetime of friendship and years of conversations over good food and wine.

Caroline Batchelder, for the tedious (but now not thankless) task of creating the index.

My family: Alison for traipsing with me across the world, leaving two adult children behind; my daughters Elanor and Laura and Alex, for encouragement to keep on with the job ('So how's the book going, Dad?' 'Finished at last!'). Laura and Alex deserve particular praise for staying behind in Sydney and coping with gas leaks and plumbers, and broken washing machines and repair men, and all the little dramas of taking care of the family home in the absence of their parents.

My readers, Denise Cooper, Erin Sessions and Trevor Stammers, for the generous gift of their time, expertise and wisdom. Thank you for saving me from infelicitous expressions and impenetrable prose, and for helping me clarify both my ideas and my language.

All these people deserve loud applause and long. They have contributed much to this book and whatever of value lies within its covers. The defects are, naturally, nobody's fault but mine, and so the catcalls and brickbats need to be directed my way.

1

Introduction

Medicine, biotechnology and the associated questions of ethics and practice are big news. Most days, major newspapers and websites carry stories of a new medical breakthrough, or some promising new line of research. But at times, the story of medicine can look like a poorly scripted soap opera in which a confusing cast of characters lurches from crisis to crisis. Doctors in the United States struggle to come to terms with the profession's complicity in capital punishment and military torture, while doctors in Syria are executed for offering treatment to 'enemy' combatants.[1] A current affairs show in Australia airs desperate pleas from the father of a dying child for the 'life-saving' treatment that the Australian government will not provide, while the Red Cross struggles to get antibiotics and bandages to refugee camps in Iraq and Jordan and Turkey. Medical scandals such as the abuse of patients in Britain's NHS, veteran affairs hospitals in the US, or nursing homes in Australia call into question the standing of medicine as a 'caring' profession.[2] The growing cost of health care in the Western world and the shift in global patterns of health and illness as a result of an ageing (and increasingly obese) population raise questions about the price wealthy nations are willing to pay for high-quality medical care and the goals of such care. These questions are, of course, heightened by the problems of inequalities in distribution of medical services both within countries (especially, but not only, in the US) and globally.[3]

1 See the harrowing account in *The New York Times* opinion piece on 19 November 2014 by Leonard S. Rubenstein and M. Zaher Sahloul, In Syria, Doctors Become the Victims http://www.nytimes.com/2014/11/20/opinion/in-syria-doctors-become-the-victims.html?_r=3 (accessed 24/11/14).

2 See, for instance: http://www.thehastingscenter.org/Bioethicsforum/Post.aspx?id=6993&blogid=140#ixzz383cWAiPW (accessed 21/07/14).

3 Lisa Sowle Cahill, *Theological Bioethics: Participation, Justice, Change* (Washington, DC: Georgetown University Press, 2005); Kendra G. Hotz and Matthew T. Mathews, *Dust and Breath: Faith, Health, and Why the Church Should Care about Both* (Grand Rapids: Eerdmans, 2012).

Other scenes in the medical melodrama are played out largely off-camera. Publicized instances of violence against doctors in Syria are examples of widespread violence against doctors and health-care workers around the world, especially in North Africa and Pakistan and Afghanistan, which go largely unreported. So, too, does the rising incidence of polio and other preventable diseases due to suspicion surrounding foreign vaccination programmes – not entirely irrational given Western governments' use of 'vaccination' and 'aid' programmes as a cover for espionage.[4] While there has been significant improvement in child and maternal health in the majority world,[5] there is still a serious lack of basic end of life care, care that would make a substantial difference to the last days of millions of people.[6] It is interesting and disturbing to reflect on biotechnology's quest for ever more sophisticated diagnostic and treatment options in light of these global realities.[7] And the discipline of bioethics, born in response to the moral outrage (rightly) generated by exposure of the abuses of medical research in the twentieth century, seems to be able to do nothing to fix it. Indeed, according to many reports, much bioethics has become a way to rationalize neglect and self-interest, and bioethicists do not show the kind of moral character – let alone courage – that we might expect from arbiters of the ethics of this key enterprise.[8] These and other issues show that medicine is searching for a clear understanding of what it is and what it's about.

In Australia, we are not immune to these questions. Medicine in Australia faces a number of pressures: an ageing population and projections of increased health-care costs; growing emphasis on sophisticated medical technologies,

4 See the US government's public commitment to not use programmes for counter-terrorist activities – and the acknowledgement that it has done so in the past, at great cost to community trust in aid agencies: http://www.theguardian.com/world/2014/may/20/cia-vaccination-programmes-counterterrorism (accessed 15/12/14).

5 See WHO update: http://www.who.int/mediacentre/factsheets/fs290/en/ (accessed 15/12/14).

6 http://www.bbc.co.uk/news/health-27661462 (accessed 03/06/14).

7 Maura Ryan, Justice and Genetics: Whose Holy Grail?, in *On Moral Medicine: Theological Perspectives in Medical Ethics*, ed. M. Therese Lysaught, et al. (Grand Rapids: Eerdmans, 2012); Cahill, *Theological Bioethics*. This is particularly apparent in the case of the recent Ebola outbreak (discussed in more detail in Chapter 2), for which, see Annette Rid and Ezekiel J. Emanuel, Ethical Considerations of Experimental Interventions in the Ebola Outbreak, *The Lancet* (2014), http://linkinghub.elsevier.com/retrieve/pii/S0140673614613155 (accessed 23/07/15).

8 According to some analyses of the discipline, this is, in fact, just what should be expected, given that bioethics has bought uncritically into the Baconian mindset that bedevils medicine. See Gerald P. McKenny, *To Relieve the Human Condition: Bioethics, Technology, and the Body* (Albany: University of New York Press, 1997).

often at the expense of patient *care*; increasing bureaucratic scrutiny and control over doctor–patient relationships and patterns of treatment and prescribing, in part driven by health-care 'efficiencies'; questions of 'conscientious objection' and the role of religious values in the provision of health care; and, of course, end of life care. If medicine hasn't lost its way, it's in serious danger of doing so.

This is a major concern, for medicine matters to us. Medicine is not just big news, it is also a big business. We invest huge resources in it – time, money, people, technology, infrastructure, education and training – and the emotional investment that goes along with it. Some of us spend our lives practising it. And we expect something from all of that, some 'bang' for our collective 'buck'. But there's the rub. We know something of the 'buck', the cost of medicine and the science and technology that sustain it. But just what is the 'bang' we should expect? What kinds of things can we rightly expect medicine to deliver? What are the goals of this rich and complex practice, and how might an understanding of those goals help us get to grips with the nature of the crises that beset it and how they might be resolved? For that matter, how might we see and bring into the light of public conversation other concerns – be it acute crisis or chronic malaise – that are currently hidden from our gaze? But surely, to understand what we can legitimately count as the goals or ends of medicine, we need some understanding of what medicine *is*.

Now, perhaps these are misguided questions. Perhaps some of our confusion comes from our failure to recognize that there is no one thing we can call 'medicine', just a disparate set of practices and institutions that, for the sake of convenience, we cover with a single label. There is research science in (human) biology, pharmacology, and so on. There are nursing homes and aged care facilities. There are rural hospitals and local clinics. There are general practices and medical centres. There are diagnostic laboratories and radiology departments, and so on and so forth. But there is no thing we can call 'medicine'.

If this is the case, there can, of course, be no coherent set of ends or purposes of medicine (for there is no such thing as 'medicine' to which those goals could be assigned). Perhaps, indeed, if we break down the institutions and practices that are covered by this convenient label, we might find that some or all of them have no clear form or goal. Nursing homes serve to provide care for those who are unable to care for themselves; but they also serve to generate

Does "medicine" have a purpose?
Is there such a thing as "medicine"?

income for their operators, provide a safe place for people to leave their relatives with a more-or-less clear conscience, and a convenient way for us as a society to avert our eyes from the frailties and indignities of disability, age and approaching death. Plastic surgery serves to correct the disfiguring effects of injury, surgery or bad genetic luck; but it also serves to allow people to sculpt their bodies to their ideal form, providing the 'perfection' that Nature denied them or age threatens to erode, as well as generating a major industry and great wealth for successful operators.

These are some of the questions I want to explore philosophically and theologically. Here is where my argument is headed. For all the complexity and diversity of the institutions and practices that make it up, I contend that there is such a thing as 'medicine'. And it has, or should have, a coherent set of goals or ends that ought to govern it as a practice. Furthermore, Christian faith, and the philosophical and theological resources with which it provides us, helps us to think well about the nature and goals of medicine, as well as providing some challenging suggestions as to how we should view it and what it should be about. The results of this inquiry are both surprising and contentious, for I am not persuaded that the standard view that medicine is *about* health and healing and the alleviation of suffering works, despite its currency in both popular and academic treatments of medicine.[9] I am not making the (wildly implausible) claim that medicine has nothing to do with health or the alleviation of suffering; my claim is that health and healing and the alleviation of suffering adequately describe neither the primary goal of medicine nor its nature. Such a claim will require justification. That, along with establishing how I think we should view the nature and goals of medicine, is what the rest of this book aims to do. Medicine, I will claim, is primarily an expression of care for vulnerable human beings whose finitude and frailty has been exposed by physical or psychological ailment and whose ability to function in meaningful relationships has been compromised; its goal is to care for such vulnerable people so as to demonstrate our solidarity with them as suffering persons and seek to enable them to return

[9] See, for instance, Edmund D. Pellegrino and David C. Thomasma, *Helping and Healing: Religious Commitment in Health Care* (Washington, DC: Georgetown University Press, 1997) and the important Hastings Center Report, Specifying the Goals of Medicine, *Hastings Center Report* 26, no. 6 (1996). While both have very helpful discussions of the nature and goals of medicine, they also both focus on health and healing, and the Hastings Center Report outlines four goals of medicine with little attempt to outline a coherent view of what medicine *is*.

to a reasonable level of functioning in relationships. Theologically, medicine is an appropriate expression of a well-formed community's care for vulnerable members of the community, a reflection of the character of God and an anticipation of the final transformation of all things to which God is drawing us and all things.

Now let me be clear: this is a book on philosophy and theology of medicine, it is not a book on bioethics. I'm not sure that the world needs another book on bioethics: along with studies on the theology of Paul or the historical Jesus or the theology of Karl Barth, bioethics has generated a volume of literature that by itself justifies Ecclesiastes' weary words: 'Of making many books there is no end, much study is a weariness of the flesh' (Eccl. 12:12, ESV). In comparison, the literature on philosophy and medicine, and especially *theology* and medicine, is much slighter (and a little less wearisome). I will refer to bioethics literature, but only where it touches on these broader questions relating to the nature and purpose of medicine.

I will also draw on a number of theological discussions of medicine. While useful, they generally have a different focus to mine. Many provide a theological framework for or grounding of a specific ethics of medicine or bioethics more generally. These normally focus on questions of human dignity and the theological anthropology (doctrine of humanity) that undergirds answers to the questions of human worth and the goal and limits of medical care.[10] Others focus on the nature of healing, divine and human, and the role that medicine might play in that.[11] These works do not do quite the task I have set myself, as medicine is more than bioethics and is both more and other than healing. Furthermore, framing the discussion in terms of healing also introduces matters such as God as the true source of all healing, whether that be 'miraculous' or 'natural' (better, the result of God's providential ordering of and action in created structures), connections between 'spirituality' (whatever that

10 See, for instance, the discussions in Megan Best, *Fearfully and Wonderfully Made: Ethics and the Beginning of Human Life* (Sydney: Matthias Media, 2012); George Khushf, Illness, the Problem of Evil, and the Analogical Structure of Healing: On the Difference Christianity Makes in Bioethics, *Christian Bioethics* 1, no. 1 (1995); James Rusthoven, *Covenantal Biomedical Ethics for Contemporary Medicine: An Alternative to Principles-Based Ethics* (Eugene, OR: Pickwick, 2014); John Wyatt, *Matters of Life and Death: Human Dilemmas in the Light of the Christian Faith* (Nottingham: IVP, 2009).

11 See, for instance, Daniel E. Fountain, *Health, the Bible and the Church* (Wheaton: Billy Graham Centre, 1989); Khushf, Illness, the Problem of Evil, and the Analogical Structure of Healing, 102–120; W. Meredith Long, *Health, Healing and God's Kingdom* (Oxford: Regnum, 2000).

is) and medicine, and so on. While these matters are all theologically interesting, they are only tangentially related to questions of what medicine is (as a human practice not a work of divine agency) and what it is for (as an immanent project, not an eschatological achievement). And so my focus will be on philosophical and theological questions related to the nature and goals of medicine.

While I'm doing a little preliminary ground-clearing, let me make some observations about the nature of philosophy and theology. While they are clearly different disciplines, they are crucially related, such that the boundaries between them for a Christian philosopher-theologian are blurry at best. This is necessarily the case, as philosophy is best understood as 'thinking carefully (and critically) about things that matter'; and so there may be a particular body of philosophical literature, but it is neither quarantined from nor oblivious to broader questions of life. Indeed, the point of philosophy is to think well about important questions. Many of those questions relate to transcendent goods, ends and values; they deal with fundamental metaphysical questions relating to the nature of humanity, community, even the value of the physical universe and of God's engagement in it – all questions which are also theology's brief. And in as much as theology ought to think carefully and critically about its subject, it will use the tools of philosophical analysis in its analytical and constructive work – or at least the tools of theology will look remarkably like the tools of philosophy and be used in similar ways.[12] So, sometimes what I call 'philosophy' of medicine may seem overly theological; at other times, what I call 'theology' of medicine may seem to be driven by philosophical concerns. That is not the result of a lack of rigour; it is due to the nature of the enterprise, the permeable boundaries between philosophy and theology, and the way that an integrated Christian view of the world and how we live in it ought to work.

So, the particular task I have set myself is to try to think carefully and critically about the nature and goals of medicine, and to do so in light of the wisdom of philosophy and the insights of Scripture and the Christian tradition.

12 Here, I betray my commitment to particular traditions of both theology and philosophy. As will become clear, I work broadly in the tradition of neo-Calvinist philosophy and theology, and have been influenced mainly by those working in the analytical philosophical tradition, most particularly Nicholas Wolterstorff. See Nicholas Wolterstorff, *Reason within the Bounds of Religion*, 2nd edn. (Grand Rapids: Eerdmans, 1984); *Until Justice and Peace Embrace* (Grand Rapids: Eerdmans, 1983).

This brings me back to what I think medicine is *not* and what it is *not* about. First, as I mentioned earlier, medicine is not about healing, or improving health. It is true that modern medicine has made extraordinary advances in understanding and treating diseases, and most of us have benefited from them (indeed, many of us are still alive because of them): germ theory and antibiotics; asepsis, pain management and anaesthesia and surgery; epidemiology and public health; the list goes on. However, at a population level, medicine is neither an efficient improver of health, nor is it primarily responsible for the dramatic improvements in health and longevity seen in the 'developing' world. Decent public policy and infrastructure, stable and safe social and political and economic systems, a reasonable level of education and basic social services, including public health and health education, are much more effective in improving population health, as is evident historically. Furthermore, seeing medicine as being about 'healing' creates insuperable problems for much of our practice, especially in relation to disability, chronic illness and the care of the dying. So one popular notion of what medicine is and is about won't do.

An obvious alternative is to see medicine as being about alleviating suffering. However, this is equally unsatisfactory. Again, some clear instances of what we would normally count as crucial medical practices illuminate this claim. First, there are many conditions that are the proper focus of medical care but which do not (directly) cause people suffering: maternal and early childhood health, hypertension and obesity, and so on. Second, there are circumstances in which people clearly suffer, but their suffering can at best be ameliorated, not removed; chronic pain and terminal illness are clear examples. Despite the growing belief that in such circumstances medicine ought to end people's suffering, even if it entails ending their life, that has not been how medicine has seen itself, and it is not how most Christians would see it. The old medical cliché reminds us of this: cure sometimes, relieve often, care always.

Now, let me be clear: health and healing and the alleviating of suffering are certainly medical concerns (as the cliché shows). My claim is not that medicine has nothing to do with them; of course it does. My claim is that these are not what medicine is about; they are not the best categories to help us understand what medicine is and what medicine is for. Figuring out those questions requires a bit of preliminary work in understanding what they entail and which background issues and conceptual concerns need to be addressed in order to answer them. When addressed philosophically and theologically, questions such as these go beyond mere description of the kinds of things that are called 'medicine' in the various contexts in which the term is used. They extend to normative questions such as: How *should* we think about medicine? How *should* we understand it as a complex social phenomenon? What are the *proper* ends of this practice or set of practices?

Moreover, I will be asking these questions as a Christian, and so theology will have a role in framing and answering them. For, as a Christian, I can think of no normative questions that I could ask about medicine (or anything else for that matter) that are not informed by my Christian commitment. Understandings of God, the world, human nature and community and their destiny, and so on, guide and govern my thinking about these matters; and so, the resources of the Christian tradition, most particularly the Scriptures, will be brought to bear on this analysis. While some might dispute this, believing that these matters of faith ought to be left out of the realm of public rational discourse, I don't believe that this is either desirable or possible. That is too big a claim to justify here, and I and others have done so elsewhere.[13] So, let me take that as a given for the moment, and note one last preliminary matter before I get on with providing a philosophical and theological account of the nature and goals of medicine.

While this is an attempt to think Christianly (and so philosophically and theologically) about medicine, it aims to use the tools of philosophy and theology to assist medical practitioners and others interested in medicine to think carefully about medicine and its goals. As such, I will not indulge in extensive footnotes, or attempt to give an exhaustive survey of the relevant literature, such as would be the norm for a technical work in philosophy or theology.[14] Rather, I will focus on particular exemplars, be they thinkers or particular works in the field, and attempt to analyse them and their contribution to the discussion, making judicious use of footnotes and using a minimum of technical vocabulary.

Let me now give you a brief outline of my argument. In the next chapter, I will present two contrasting stories from the 2014 Ebola outbreak that raise

13 See Andrew Sloane, *On Being a Christian in the Academy: Nicholas Wolterstorff and the Practice of Christian Scholarship* (Carlisle: Paternoster, 2003) and the literature cited there.

14 I will address some of these matters and questions related to the larger project in occasional papers and posts on: http://www.morlingcollege.com/theology-medicine

important questions about the nature and goals of medicine and help us see something of the diverse contexts in which it operates. One is the more familiar (to me) context of the Western world and the growing commodification of medicine evident in the West and the problems this generates for medicine as a moral enterprise. The other is the majority world and the difficulties those who practise medicine need to face in dealing with the scarcity of resources, and the way this highlights important issues for our understanding of and engagement in medicine as a social practice. This first entry point into the world of medicine will demonstrate both the need for careful reflection on the underlying nature of medicine and human community, as well as providing a way into the philosophy of medicine.[15]

Bioethics is another doorway into this discussion, and I will address it in Chapter 3. I will demonstrate the contested nature of bioethics, and show how bioethical debate reflects an underlying vision of humanity and society with reference to two representative issues. First, I will evaluate the key lines of argument on a contentious issue (euthanasia), showing how the arguments presented are reflective of deeper 'world-and-life-view' concerns, partially explaining the intractable nature of bioethical disagreements. Second, I will examine Janet Radcliffe Richards' discussion of a seemingly straightforward issue (the ethics of organ transplantation), showing that deeper philosophical and theological issues also are at stake in such discussions.

Chapter 4 will shift focus to directly address issues of the philosophy of medicine. I will identify a few issues that I believe are particularly pertinent to my underlying questions: What is medicine? And what is it for? I will begin with a discussion of the concept of health, seeking to understand both what health is (a surprisingly tricky question) and what its connection to medicine might be. I will then change tack, looking at the movement known as 'evidence-based medicine' in order to figure out how it sees medicine and particularly medical knowing (epistemology) and the problems this generates. The chapter will close with a discussion of the phenomenology of illness and the clinical

15 It is interesting to note that consideration of the social context/s of medicine as an initial and framing concern is something of an innovation in bioethics, but one that rightly is seen to reconfigure the discussion. See M. Therese Lysaught et al. (eds.), *On Moral Medicine: Theological Perspectives in Medical Ethics*, 3rd edn. (Grand Rapids: Eerdmans, 2012), 117–119, the editor's introduction to Part II, Christianity and the Social Practice of Health Care, and also the discussion of US and global issues on pp.162–164.

encounter, seeking to articulate what it might demonstrate about central experiences and practices related to medicine and medical practice.

In Chapter 5, I will move to specifically theological questions. The chapter will open with an account of recent critiques of the culture of medicine from both Catholic and Protestant perspectives. While I do not agree that there is a single, coherent tradition of medical practice that has become eroded in modern technical medicine, some important insights can be drawn from this work. This will lead me to an examination of the work of Stanley Hauerwas, one of the more acute critics of the way that modern medicine is a truly *modern* enterprise: it seeks to overcome the limitations and frailties of human existence in light of a false narrative of modernity. While there are problems with both his analysis of medicine and his proposal for its remedy, he has important insights from which we must learn. I will close with a discussion of the explicitly Christian philosophy of medicine articulated by Edmund Pellegrino and David Thomasma, noting its insightful analysis of the clinical encounter, as well as the flaws in the theological and philosophical frameworks that inform their work.

Chapter 6 will consist of something of a necessary detour into the theology of health, drawing on the recent work of Neil Messer. Messer argues that we need a clear understanding of the notion of health (both what it does and does not mean) if we are to have a proper grounding for a theology of health care and a theological bioethics. He draws this from the work of Karl Barth and Thomas Aquinas (not normally seen as comfortable theological bed-fellows), placing his account of health in the context of an understanding of human flourishing that is both teleological (goal-oriented) and eschatological (relating to the way that God will bring all things to God's desired goal in the end). Again, there is much to learn from his work: nonetheless, the very clarity of his discussion demonstrates the inherently 'fuzzy' nature of 'health' and points us towards its inadequacy as a framing notion for the practice of medicine. He, somewhat ironically perhaps, shows that 'health and healing' do not satisfactorily account for the nature and goals of medicine.

Chapter 7 will, I suppose, be yet a further detour into general theological territory, providing what I believe to be two necessary frameworks for an adequate account of medicine. The first deals with the nature of knowledge and of scholarship (epistemology). I will draw on recent work in the theory of knowledge to outline a perspective on human belief-formation that accents the personal, particular, contextual and embodied nature of human knowledge, but which also acknowledges that, when properly governed, our attempts to understand ourselves and the world aim at attaining the truth of the matter, however elusive that may be. This will, I believe, help us understand medicine as a practice of inquiry and the bodies of knowledge it generates (with apologies for the entirely intentional pun). The second is a biblical-theological 'grand narrative' that provides the context and framework for Christian theological reflection on matters such as medicine. It seeks to understand medicine in light of a coherent theological account of reality, including the nature of human community, which serves to inform our concept of medicine, its limits, goals and role in God's grand programme of transforming a broken world and broken creatures that are yet of inestimable value to God.

In Chapter 8, I will, at last, outline what I take to be the nature and goals of medicine. I will discuss this from a number of points of view, seeking to pick up the insights of the previous argument, as well as bringing to bear further conceptual tools. One important analytical tool is MacIntyre's notion of a 'social practice' and his understanding of virtue as a set of 'excellences' associated with the attaining of the goods that are internal to that practice. This notion has provided insight into medicine and other complex social phenomena, and serves to elucidate both the nature and goals of medicine and its intrinsically moral character. Returning again to the notion of health, and the problems associated with it, I will close this chapter with a discussion of human vulnerability and finitude and the nature of medicine. My central claim is that medicine is best understood as an expression of a good community's 'standing with' those of its number whose ability to function well in the community is disrupted as a result of physical or psychological frailty. The goal of this enterprise is to care for vulnerable creatures. One form that care may take is to seek to combat illness and disease and/or return people to 'health'; but that is not the only form it takes. Its primary goal is to express that solidarity with others in their embodied vulnerability that is required of a properly functioning human community. But it also recognizes the clear limits placed on that enterprise, like all human enterprises, by the very nature of human finitude. This appropriately chastens medicine and the goals it sets itself, and provides a framework within which to address the questions of appropriate care, resource distribution, bioethical dilemmas, and so on with which I opened the book.

The final chapter, then, will bring the argument together and to bear on those questions I raised at the beginning of this discussion. I will seek to show that the understanding of medicine I have articulated helps us analyse issues such as euthanasia or organ transplantation, providing an essential context in which to address these and other bioethical issues. I will also show how it helps us understand questions such as what constitutes appropriate care (and levels of care) in the widely variable contexts we find in the world. I will close with some reflections on how this vision might inform a doctor's self-understanding, and how it might inform the training of prospective doctors.

2

Entering the World of Medicine – Contexts

Introduction: learning from a tragedy

Medicine is a strange enterprise and an uncomfortable one. One of the stranger and more uncomfortable features of the discipline is the way that tragedy is the theatre of learning. This is so familiar to doctors as to be almost invisible. We learn anatomy in the dissecting room – using the exposed corpse of another human being, someone whose exit from the world left a hole in the lives of their family and friends, to understand and manipulate the human body. We learn pathology in the laboratory and at the bedside of the sick and dying – using their illnesses and the effects of disease on tissues and bodily functions to understand disease processes and their causes and possible cures. We learn epidemiology by studying epidemics – using the spread of diseases through communities and the trail of death and disability they leave behind to understand their effects on human populations. This is all a matter of course for doctors but is strange and uncomfortable for those who have not been inducted by these methods into the practice of medicine. One of my aims in this book is to encourage doctors to think about this strange and uncomfortable enterprise, seeing afresh something of its oddness, gaining a little clinical distance, so to speak, from their immersion in their everyday practice to help them think about what they are doing and why. But before I get to that, I want to use the patterns of medical knowing on medicine. That is to say, I want to use a current tragedy as a theatre of learning about medicine and where it finds itself in the world.

Medicine is often in the headlines. In the West, those headlines are normally about 'us': questions of medicine in the West such as end of life care or the latest medical breakthrough (or its unavailability to a photogenic sufferer of a tragic condition). In 2014, Western issues were pushed out of the headlines by a disease few had heard of until then, and none were likely to suffer: Ebola. I want to see what we can learn about medicine from the Ebola epidemic in West Africa. This is not, I hope, to trivialize it, or voyeuristically subject it to our inquisitive gaze, or just to see it as something useful to my purposes. That, of course, can happen when learning from tragedy, as evidenced by abuses of anatomical specimens in medical schools and those egregious abuses of experimental subjects that prompted the rise of bioethics.[1] We need to recognize the human tragedies that lie behind our learning and respect those who have paid the price of our instruction both in how we gain knowledge and how we use it – which entails doing what we can to deal with the disease. Nonetheless, learn from it we must. So, let me tell the stories of two doctors: Kent Brantly and Sheik Umar Khan and their contrasting fates; Brantly's eventual recovery after medical evacuation to the US, and Khan's succumbing to the disease in Sierra Leone. In doing so, I cast no aspersions on their respective organizations, nor is there any element of blame. Nonetheless, their differing fates do illustrate aspects of the contrasting contexts of medicine in the West and the majority world that we would do well to examine.

As is now well known, Kent Brantly is an American doctor who worked with Samaritan's Purse in West Africa during the Ebola epidemic and survived the disease after treatment at the Emory University Hospital in Atlanta, Georgia. Dr Brantly received his training in medicine at Indiana University, graduating in 2009. Soon after qualifying, he joined the Christian mission and relief agency Samaritan's Purse and was deployed to Liberia to engage in medical care and relief in October 2013, prior to the outbreak of Ebola in West Africa. When the disease spread to Liberia in June 2014, he was one of two doctors engaged in the care of people with the Ebola virus. Despite due diligence, he contracted the disease in Liberia on 23 July, and after initial treatment in Monrovia was evacuated to the US, and was admitted to Emory

1 On misuse of anatomy specimens see, for instance, http://www.smh.com.au/news/national/cadaver-abuse-unsw-apologises/2007/02/06/1170524072141.html (accessed 12/03/14). For an account of the development of bioethics in response to scandals in medical research, see James Rusthoven, *Covenantal Biomedical Ethics for Contemporary Medicine: An Alternative to Principles-Based Ethics* (Eugene, OR: Pickwick, 2014), 13–47.

University Hospital on 2 August 2014. After receiving sophisticated medical care, much of it unavailable in Monrovia, and the controversial and experimental drug ZMapp, he made a full recovery and was discharged on 21 August 2014.[2]

As is, perhaps, less well known, Sheik Umar Khan was a Sierra Leonean doctor who worked with the ministry of health in Sierra Leone during the Ebola epidemic and succumbed to the disease on 29 July 2014. Dr Khan received his training in medicine at the College of Medicine and Allied Health Sciences of the University of Sierra Leone in Freetown, graduating in 2001. Soon after qualifying, he began working on infectious diseases in West Africa, focusing on haemorrhagic fevers such as Lassa fever. He was integral to the medical response to the growing Ebola epidemic in Sierra Leone, working with both the government and international agencies such as the World Health Organization (WHO) and Médecins Sans Frontières (MSF). Despite being aware of the risks of contracting the disease and being urged to leave the risks to others, he continued to work in trying conditions with limited resources, both caring for infected patients and seeking to implement strategies to limit the spread of the disease. He was, by all accounts, careful to maintain standards of hygiene and infection control, but became infected with the virus, testing positive on 22 July 2014. There was some initial improvement in his condition, prompting those treating him to hope that he might recover. Tragically, he rapidly deteriorated and died from the disease on 29 July at the Ebola Treatment Centre in Kailahun.[3] His death is one of many personal tragedies caused by this epidemic. Since the outbreak began in late 2013, an estimated 15,351 people have been infected and 5,459 people have died, most with limited access to health care.[4]

So, that is the tragedy. But where is the learning? What does this teach us about medicine in our world today?

2 See http://www.samaritanspurse.org/article/samaritans-purse-doctor-recovered-from-ebola/; http://inscopearchive.iu.edu/headlines/2014-07-30-headline-brantley-statement-inscope.shtml; http://edition.cnn.com/2014/08/02/health/ebola-kent-brantly/; http://time.com/3270016/ebola-survivor-kent-brantly/ (accessed 26/11/14).

3 For this, and other details of his career, see the BBC report of his death, http://www.bbc.com/news/world-africa-28560507 (accessed 26/11/14).

4 Figures current at the time of writing. See http://www.who.int/csr/disease/ebola/situation-reports/en/ (accessed 26/11/14).

The global context of medicine

Perhaps the most obvious set of questions relates to the kinds of treatment that are available in different contexts and the resources required to establish and maintain and deploy them. I will begin where the media often does: the use of experimental treatments. One striking feature of these contrasting stories is that ZMapp, the experimental anti-viral agent successfully used to treat Brantly, was available for the treatment of Khan, but was rejected on ethical grounds.[5] Again, I'm not making judgements about either the ethics of that decision (which was carefully considered by his treating physicians), nor about the possible efficacy of the treatment (since Miguel Pajares and Abraham Borbor both died, though treated with the drug).[6] In many respects, these decisions are common in the resource-rich Western medical system. Whether the decision relates to a new, experimental chemotherapeutic agent for malignancy, or genetic therapies for rare conditions,[7] or a complex and lengthy and risky surgical procedure, in a context such as mine in Australia, decisions like that, while difficult, are almost commonplace. The decision not to use ZMapp on Khan and to use it on Brantly were, to a great extent, decisions made on clinical and ethical grounds.[8] No such decisions are foolproof; medical knowing is not the kind of knowing that brings that sort of certainty. Judgement is always needed, and judgements can always be disputed.

My point, rather, is that their different treatment reflects the disparities in medical services available to patients in the Western and majority worlds, and the disparities in the resources available to treat them. So more important than the question of whether Brantly or Khan did or did not receive ZMapp is the question of where these decisions were made and in what kind of medical context. Khan was treated – and treated well, no doubt – at the Ebola Treatment Centre in Kailahun, a field hospital in Sierra Leone; after his initial care

[5] See http://www.cbc.ca/news/health/dying-sierra-leone-dr-sheik-umar-khan-never-told-ebola-drug-was-available-1.2738163 (accessed 26/11/14).

[6] Miguel Pajares was a Spanish priest who died in hospital in Madrid; Abraham Borbor was a Liberian doctor who died in hospital in Monrovia. See http://www.theguardian.com/world/2014/oct/01/first-ebola-patient-us-no-zmapp (accessed 26/11/14).

[7] See, for instance, http://www.reuters.com/article/2014/11/26/us-health-genetherapy-price-idUSKCN0JA1TP20141126 (accessed 27/11/14).

[8] Given the involvement of MSF, I think it highly unlikely that Khan's ethnicity or national origin were factors in the decision not to use the drug.

(including the dose of ZMapp), Brantly was treated – and treated well, no doubt – at Emory University Hospital, a tertiary teaching hospital in the US. The diagnostic and therapeutic resources available at these institutions differ more than many of us used to the practice of medicine in the West can imagine. Emory is a familiar environment to those of us accustomed to Western technological medicine. More-or-less state of the art equipment, ready access to a wide range of investigations (biochemical, microbiological, imaging, and so forth) and treatment options including, where needed, intravenous fluids and blood products, circulatory support, artificial ventilation, and so on. In short, the kind of facilities available to patients in an early twenty-first century ICU in a tertiary medical centre. Having been evacuated from Sierra Leone to the US, all of these facilities were available for the treatment of Brantly and, whatever the effects of ZMapp, the ability to closely monitor and support him physiologically in the acute phase of the illness was crucial to his survival. Little, if any, of this was available to Khan in the field hospital in Sierra Leone. This was not due to malice or neglect on the behalf of those treating him. It was due, quite simply, to the exigencies of his being treated in a field hospital in West Africa. Medical resources are stretched to breaking point and beyond. Even if samples could be taken and equipment be made available, the institutional framework that makes them *useful* – even deployable – did not exist. The close monitoring used in Brantly's treatment requires well-equipped laboratory and radiology facilities and the staff and materials needed to use them. The intensive medical treatment and support used in his care requires well-equipped medical facilities and a large and well-trained staff and a great deal of *materiel* in order to be effective. Despite the best will in the world, such facilities are unavailable, and cannot reasonably be expected to be available, in a context such as the Ebola Treatment Centre in Kailahun. This lack of medical resources clearly has deleterious consequences for patients in those areas. But it does not, in fact, require very sophisticated services to make a substantial difference in these conditions of great need and great want: for very often, significant gains can be made through relatively simple 'supportive' measures such as intravenous hydration. While it seems unreasonable to expect everyone to have access to a tertiary treatment centre, it does not seem unreasonable to expect everyone to have access to a level of care that would support them in their illness. Such supportive care may, in fact, be enough to see them through the crisis; it may not. At the very least, however, it seems such care is a basic expression of our commitment to suffering people at risk of death or serious disability.

And so, while the focus has generally been on the use of ZMapp for particular high-profile patients, it seems to me that we need to pay more attention to the questions of context, resources and institutional frameworks that make decisions in some circumstances even imaginable, and decisions in others impossible. Choices that we in the West take for granted are unimaginable in many other medical contexts. These raise profound questions about the nature and goals of medicine, and we need to wrestle with these questions.[9] For if medicine is about fighting disease and forestalling death, then those who treated Brantly succeeded in their task, while those who treated Khan failed. But it seems odd to conclude that the extraordinary efforts made to treat suffering people in West Africa are medical *failures* in the sixty per cent or so of cases in which the patient dies.[10] On the other hand, if medicine is about improving the health of people and communities, then *both* cases must count as failures. For Khan died (and so obviously his medical care did not improve his health); and the treatment centre deals only with those who succumb to the disease, rather than dealing with the circumstances that allow for its spread through a population.[11] Equally, while Brantly recovered, this came at considerable cost in time, money, personnel and *materiel*, a cost that cannot reasonably be borne for all who suffer from Ebola, Lassa fever, cerebral malaria, or other endemic diseases. And clearly, an equivalent amount of time, money, personnel and *materiel*, if deployed in, say, public health or the development of

[9] I will examine these questions in Chapter 9. For preliminary reflections, see Andrew Sloane, Painful Justice: An Ethical Perspective on the Allocation of Trauma Services in Australia, *The Australian and New Zealand Journal of Surgery* 68, no. 11 (1998); Christianity and the Transformation of Medicine, in *Christianity and the Disciplines: The Transformation of the University*, ed. Oliver D. Crisp et al. (London: T&T Clark, 2012), 85–87, 93.

[10] Please note: I am claiming that healing is not the best way of understanding what they were about, not that they didn't understand their goal in treating Khan as restoring him to health. I will return to this question later, but for now let me say again: health and healing are important elements in the practice of medicine, but they do not give us a satisfactory framework for understanding its essential nature or its primary goals. This is evident in these instances, and perhaps more obviously in 'pre-modern' medicine which had limited resources to either cure disease or ease suffering, and yet must, I would suggest, be counted as a legitimate instance of medical practice lest we fall prey to the most egregious excesses of temporal snobbery.

[11] On the role of basic health care and public health measures in the Ebola crisis, see: Annette Rid and Ezekiel J. Emanuel, Ethical Considerations of Experimental Interventions in the Ebola Outbreak, *The Lancet* (2014), http://linkinghub.elsevier.com/retrieve/pii/S0140673614613155; http://www.bioedge.org/index.php/bioethics/bioethics_article/11104 (accessed 15/12/14).

physical and social infrastructure, would have considerably greater impact on the health and well-being of affected communities.[12]

Now these are important questions in their own right. My point, however, is not that the care offered to either Brantly or Khan was inappropriate (far from it, as I will discuss shortly). My point is that these questions point to other, deeper questions about the nature and goals of medicine. If the categories and questions we typically use to assess medicine and its 'success' lead to such problematic conclusions, it may be that we're using the wrong categories and asking the wrong questions. It also shows us that medical care, important as it is, is not the most important factor in saving lives. In the case of Ebola, effective public health and quarantine measures would do more to slow the spread of disease and limit new cases than any amount of acute medical care.[13] Furthermore, these primarily social policy and civil infrastructure measures would have impact far beyond crises such as Ebola. It is estimated that nine per cent of the global disease burden could be reduced simply by providing access to clean water and decent sanitation.[14] Similarly, the recent dramatic decrease in the incidence of malaria and associated suffering and death is largely the result of the provision of mosquito nets and insecticides – hardly medical treatments.[15] But, such public health, sanitation and quarantine measures are impossible without a high level of social stability, infrastructure, public education, and so forth. So, once again, if health is not in any straightforward way the point of medicine or what justifies its existence, we return to the questions: What *is* medicine? And what is it *for*?

The state of Western medicine

These stories, and the way the epidemic has been portrayed in the media and handled by government and other agencies, also tell us something important about the social and cultural contexts in which medicine is practised. A

12 A point made with great force in the public health literature. See, for instance, Fran Baum, *The New Public Health*, 3rd edn. (South Melbourne: Oxford University Press, 2008).

13 At the time of writing, these measures seem to be taking effect, with a reduction in new cases of Ebola in Liberia and to a lesser extent in Sierra Leone. See http://www.bbc.com/news/world-africa-28755033; http://www.cdc.gov/vhf/ebola/; http://www.who.int/csr/disease/ebola/situation-reports/en/ (accessed 26/11/14).

14 http://www.cdc.gov/healthywater/global/wash_statistics.html (accessed 05/12/14).

15 See http://www.bbc.com/news/health-30375202 (accessed 11/12/14).

number of observations come to mind. The first is the almost panicked reaction in Western nations. I was particularly struck, I must say, by the reaction in my homeland, Australia. We are, perhaps, the nation most 'quarantined' from the risk of Ebola, due to geographical isolation, relatively limited lines of contact with West African communities, and a reasonably efficient and effective hospital and public health system. And yet both media reports and initial government in/action suggested that we were in imminent danger of a catastrophic epidemic, such that sending Australian personnel to assist in the international response would be irresponsible.

At first glance, this response is puzzling – perhaps just another expression of the florid xenophobia that seems to be infecting politics in Australia (and other wealthy nations). But further reflection suggests that something deeper is going on, something to do with our expectations of medicine and public health and the way we conduct our lives. For there is no such panicked response to outbreaks of malaria (including multiple drug-resistant forms), or to epidemics of infectious diarrhoea, despite the fact that they are the leading causes of death from infectious diseases in the world. And that, I suggest, is because we do not feel vulnerable to those threats. Perhaps we realize that the primary disease vectors (the Anopheles mosquito, for instance) do not threaten us (unless we live in the tropical far north of the country); or we recognize that we can take precautions that are likely to protect us from infection (using mosquito nets and DEET, or careful hand-washing and eating habits); or we believe that we will receive treatment that will cure us of the disease should we catch it (fluids and antibiotics or anti-malarials). Unlike most people through most of human history – and, for that matter, most people in the world today – we in the West simply do not expect to die of infectious diseases. We expect that there will be a drug of some sort that will cure us, that medicine can fix what ails us (which, of course, also explains the frequent tabloid reports of new 'super-bugs', pathogens resistant to available pharmaceutical agents). We no longer see ourselves as vulnerable to the accidents of history, the vicissitudes of time and place that constrain our lives and may even cut them short. Such expectations are both the product of the successes of modern medicine and also shape its practice and the expectations we have of it, for good and for ill.

However, we also expect that doctors will treat sick people, whether there is a chance for a cure or not – and sometimes at great personal cost, even risk to the doctor's life, as the care that both Brantly and Khan gave and received demonstrates. We need to think about the virtues of medical practice: for both men risked their lives in order to care for sick and vulnerable people ... But is that right? Is what they did obligatory or supererogatory – a morally praiseworthy commitment, but not one required of doctors?[16] Or is it an expression of paradoxical selfishness, a willingness for others to be coerced into rescuing them when their risky behaviour leads to harm? Perhaps the distinction between moral 'saints' and moral 'heroes' might help us?[17] Western culture tends to value moral 'heroes', those who put their lives on the line in crisis situations and, whatever their personal qualities, perform some great good. Their impact is obvious, and often public, but generally fleeting, and leaves us in awe. Moral 'saints', on the other hand, are those who by way of the everyday conduct of their lives and the general shape of their moral endeavours seek to do good and be good and so make a difference in the world. Often, their impact is noticed only when their presence is gone and the great benefits they brought are missed, but their influence on our lives and communities endures, and leaves us better people. Few of us can aspire to being either moral saints or moral heroes (indeed, by its very nature, heroism is not something we can aim at, but something we fall into – or not). Medical morality is best understood, I would suggest, under the category of moral 'saintliness' rather than moral heroism; it is a matter of the general conduct of a life and the goods we seek to achieve. What, then, of the seemingly heroic actions of those like Brantly and Khan who risk their lives in the service of others, and what kind of care do we owe them?

Let me make some preliminary observations, in anticipation of a more complete discussion in the final chapter. It seems to me that there is an implicit obligation laid on the rest of us to care for those prepared to take personal risks to help others 'above and beyond' ordinary care. This is not just the product of the utilitarian value of that care (that is, such care has more 'bang for buck' than care for others because of their potential benefit to the sick). Nor is it a

16 For contrasting perspectives on this question, see Rusthoven, *Covenantal Biomedical Ethics*, 241–271; Tom L. Beauchamp and James F. Childress, *Principles of Biomedical Ethics*, 7th edn. (Oxford: Oxford University Press, 2008), 202–214.

17 For this useful distinction, see Samuel Wells, *Improvisation: The Drama of Christian Ethics* (Grand Rapids: Brazos, 2004), esp. 42–44.

reward for costly service. Rather, special care for those who engage in risky care for others is best understood as a way of fostering the kind of commitment required of those who engage in the practice of medicine, and an expression of the underlying rationale of medical care. That is, 'risky' care is a way of expressing solidarity with sick and vulnerable people rather than abandoning them; caring for those who are willing to risk themselves to care for others is required both because it is itself an expression of solidarity with the (newly) sick, and because that care is an indirect expression of solidarity with the vulnerable, as it signals the lengths we will go to care for those who are our 'hands and feet' in those circumstances. Of course, it only makes sense as an expression of a broader vision of community in which we recognize that our responsibilities to the vulnerable, while not boundless, are nonetheless extensive. These are not, I would think, virtues specific to medical practice, but are specific medical expressions of those virtues that constitute proper moral character in godly human community.

This relates to the contested question of the virtues of medical practice and the extent to which they are unique to medicine or are particular forms of more general virtues (I would suggest the latter). But in as much as medical care is an embodiment (so to speak) of our communal commitment to solidarity to the vulnerable rather than their abandonment, these are obligations that fall particularly on medical practitioners. And, I daresay, most particularly on *Christian* medical practitioners. This is not because only Christians are called to exhibit the virtues, values and actions of godly community, but because our call is to exemplify the forms of proper human community now enabled by the freedom that is ours in Christ and the life-giving power of the Spirit.

There are other issues that are particular to a context of plenty, such as in Western countries like Australia. Everyone who has worked in a Western hospital system would be familiar with difficult decisions relating to the diagnosis and treatment of complex cases (some of which have been alluded to earlier). A bewildering array of investigations is available – biochemical, haematological, serological, bacteriological and imaging – all designed to pin down precisely what's going on with this patient. A similar array of treatment options may be available – pharmaceuticals, surgery (be it classical 'open' surgery or endoscopic or image-controlled), chemotherapy, radiotherapy, and so forth – all designed to try to treat the underlying condition. Even when 'curative' options have been exhausted and 'there's nothing more to be done', there are decisions to be made about which resources should be brought to bear in caring for this person. While there may be significant debates about the kinds of care that might be most appropriate in particular cases,[18] these debates take place in a context of a (relative) abundance of medical resources and the options they make possible and imaginable (and, for that matter, those options they render invisible or unimaginable).

The abundance of options is, I think, generally to be welcomed.[19] But we need to recognize that it is the product of particular circumstances in human history and culture, and brings with it a range of problems and questions that warrant more careful consideration. While the economic and technological conditions that make modern medicine possible are interesting and important, my focus is on philosophy and theology of medicine, and so I will explore the matters that seem more relevant to those concerns. Doing that requires telling something of the story of modern medicine. I will use two complementary accounts: Jeffrey Bishop's critical theoretical account (influenced by the work of French philosopher Michel Foucault) and Gerald McKenny's analysis of the scientific-technical rationality of 'Baconian' medicine.

Bishop seeks to understand the epistemology of medicine and its associated metaphysics in relation to Foucault's categories of 'biopolitics' and the corresponding understanding of space.[20] Bishop argues that fundamental to the practice of modern medicine is a *metaphysics* (not just an epistemology) of efficient causation.[21] That is, because immanent sequences of cause and effect can be observed – and more particularly *measured* – these sequences, and the

[18] See the discussion in Chapter 9.

[19] But see below for some significant caveats.

[20] Jeffrey P. Bishop, Foucauldian Diagnostics: Space, Time, and the Metaphysics of Medicine, *Journal of Medicine and Philosophy* 34, no. 4 (2009). 'Biopolitics' speaks of the relationship between biological sciences, the understandings of the human body that they generate, and the way they are conditioned by and foster particular forms of social organization and power relationships. 'Biopower' speaks particularly of the relationship between knowledge claims and forms of knowledge exhibited by modern medicine and the patterns of social power and control associated with them.

[21] Metaphysics (or ontology) deals with the philosophy of what exists, what kinds of things exist, and the nature of existence itself. Epistemology deals with the nature of knowledge and belief and questions to do with the nature of truth and to what extent we can attain it and under what conditions.

things that cause or are caused by them, constitute reality. Furthermore, given the essentially political nature of such measurable knowledge and the purposes to which it is put, what is real is that which is manipulable (especially, that which is subject to the controlling power of the state) and that which is observable (especially, that which is subject to the controlling observation – or 'gaze' – of the wielder of power). However, because space is primary in Foucault's understanding of 'modern' knowledge, and because biological systems are subject to change, a live body is not subject to the kind of determinative knowledge required in modernity. The dead body becomes the true 'body of knowledge' in medicine, and the basis of that knowledge which allows clinicians to manipulate live bodies for the benefit of patients.[22] As Bishop puts it:

> The static object – the dead body – and the stable subject – the dead gaze – cross one another in the clinic, where not only the bodies are totalized but also the psychosocial, and indeed the spiritual, comes to find its place in the ordering space of the clinic. The doctor, the psychiatrist, the social worker, and the hospital chaplain, all seek to manipulate bodies for the benefit of those bodies and psyches that are manipulated. Thus, by taking a Foucauldian look at medicine, one can see medicine at work, where bodies and psyches are efficiently and effectively molded, manipulated, controlled, and even coerced, by surgery, drugs, technologies, and techniques deployed by physicians, surgeons, machines, psychologists, social workers, and chaplains. The metaphysics of medicine is a metaphysics of efficient causation.[23]

This metaphysics is, he believes, both fatally flawed and not subject to cure using the resources of current medicine or bioethics. Indeed, Bishop suggests at the end of his challenging book: 'Might it not be that only theology can save medicine?'[24]

While approaching things from the perspective of bioethics and the body, similar ideas emerge from the work of Gerald McKenny on the Baconian

22 Michel Foucault, *The Birth of the Clinic: An Archaeology of Medical Perception* (New York: Vintage, 1994); see also Bishop, Foucauldian Diagnostics, esp. 344–347; *The Anticipatory Corpse: Medicine, Power and the Care of the Dying* (Notre Dame, IN: UNDP, 2011).

23 Foucauldian Diagnostics, 346–347.

24 *The Anticipatory Corpse*, 313.

tradition of modern medicine.[25] At the heart of McKenny's understanding of the Baconian project is the quest for technical mastery that will reduce or eliminate illness and suffering and limitation, and so expand the field of human choices. This entails that all suffering is, in the end, pointless, and has no meaningful role in our moral projects or the formation of us as persons. There is no overarching *telos* to human existence that enables us to understand the nature of finite and frail bodily existence or the role (and limitations) of 'health' in human flourishing. Akin to Bishop, he sees this as partly the result of modern science's exclusion of all but efficient causation and proximal ends from its explanatory frameworks, thereby eclipsing final causes or transcendent ends that might give a human life (or the cosmos, for that matter) an overarching meaning.[26] The only meanings left are immanent 'factual' explanations and the products of human will. That will is, however, an empty, 'nihilistic' will in as much as with no transcendent good towards which it ought to be oriented, the will itself becomes the only moral good to be reckoned with.[27] Technology becomes a system of power and control that we believe we use in order to further our free choices – not recognizing that technology itself inscribes systems of power on us, our bodies and our wills, such that the wills we seek to use to govern technological projects are themselves the products of them. Indeed, bodies become impediments to the exercise of choice, such that 'biopower' seeks to erase all suffering and limitations on our choices, even to the extent of eliminating the sufferer in order to eliminate their suffering.

While Bishop is clear in his analysis of the ways in which bureaucratic control distorts the care of the dying,[28] neither he nor McKenny directly address the problem of the growing commodification of medicine. This is

25 Gerald P. McKenny, *To Relieve the Human Condition: Bioethics, Technology, and the Body* (Albany: University of New York Press, 1997). Also see the excerpt Bioethics, the Body, and the Legacy of Bacon, in *On Moral Medicine: Theological Perspectives in Medical Ethics*, ed. M. Therese Lysaught et al. (Grand Rapids: Eerdmans, 2012). Francis Bacon (1561–1626) was an English philosopher and practitioner of the scientific method whose work has profoundly influenced the modernist understanding of science and development of technology.

26 Proximal, or penultimate, ends, are those that relate to tangible phenomena and our existence in history; final causes or transcendent ends relate to that which goes beyond (transcends) historical existence in relation to the divine origin of things and the eschatological (beyond history) goal of existence, including human existence.

27 See David Bentley Hart, God or Nothingness, in *I Am the Lord Your God: Christian Reflections on the Ten Commandments*, ed. Carl E. Braaten and Christopher R. Seitz (Grand Rapids: Eerdmans, 2005).

28 I will discuss the bureaucratization of medicine in Chapter 8.

particularly puzzling in McKenny's case given his focus on the Baconian quest to escape exigency and increase choice, as both elements are factors in the growth of the market ethos of late modern capitalism and its reduction of all social goods to tradeable goods – developments that clearly impact on the practice of medicine in the West. One reason for the proliferation of therapeutic options and the inability of people to turn from the quest for cure at whatever cost is just that it expands the field of choice. It is not merely that we have become blind to the realization that we are mortal, that our bodies are limited in both time and space, and so our choices and even life inevitably come to an end. It is also that medicine, as a product of technology in late modern capitalism, embodies (pun intended) the values of the cultures and economies that produce it. In this socio-economic context, 'choice' has become, if not a commodity itself, the specious rationalization for the endless expansion of products and services that fuel our societies (now reduced to economies).[29] Choice – be it lifestyle choice or available treatment options – dictates the perpetual growth of options and mandates that the only limitation on availability should be the purchasing power of the consumer. Doctors become service providers, vendors whose expertise and knowledge are available for purchase by consumers, and patients become clients or consumers, the sole arbiters of which treatment options they choose to purchase (subject, of course, to market availability).

A number of these forces come together in a growing focus on technical expertise rather than patient care. This is, in my view, reflected in diminishing emphasis on clinical skill and increasing reliance on evidence from investigations. Radiology, for instance, often focuses on getting the best images or information using the most reliable (or at least most recent) technology. This may come at the expense of effective communication with patients and reporting of results to referring doctors and even the care of patients in the department; and very often, there is little concern as to whether the information will inform patient care or change the treatment they will receive. Indeed, to

[29] For interesting reflections on the way that money distorts the practice of medicine as a profession in our capitalist context (as well as the positive uses to which it can be put), see William F. May, Money and the Medical Profession, *Kennedy Institute of Ethics Journal* 7, no. 1 (1997). For a critique of medicine as an attempt to gain mastery and expand 'choice', see Joel Shuman and Brian Volck, *Reclaiming the Body: Christians and the Faithful Use of Modern Medicine* (Grand Rapids: Brazos, 2006).

echo Bishop, this obsession with 'objective' results is either an expression of defensive medicine in the face of fear of litigation, or an instance of an 'anticipatory post-mortem', an attempt to get a definitive diagnosis for the sake of knowing what's going on rather than being concerned about the best way to care for this person.[30] Once again, these observations prompt the questions: Is this what medicine should be? Is this what medicine should be about?

The lines and lies of power and control are tangled indeed, including the interplay of technology and social vision, economics and imagination, and the ways in which they shape human volitional and corporeal existence. There is, of course, no free exercise of 'will', only the myth of autonomy as the driver of the commodification of life. We are social and economic beings; we need to become aware of the values, narratives and desires that shape us as 'agents' in a globalized marketplace. Indeed, if we are not to become inert recipients, even passive victims, of such forces, we need an alternative narrative (and the values and desires that go along with it), one that will enable us to resist these forces and express an alternative way of living in the world. Christians not only have a particular need to do so, required as we are to be 'in the world, but not of it', we also have rich resources in the Bible and our tradition that enable us to tell an alternative story and live by it, shaping and being shaped by different desires and embodying distinctive values.

These are some of the questions we must face as we consider the global context of medicine. These are not the only questions we must address; nor is this the only context that raises them. Important questions about the nature and purpose of medicine are raised by issues of bioethics, to which we now turn.

30 I will say more about medical epistemology, its nature, purpose and limits, in Chapters 4 and 7.

3

Why Bioethics Needs a Philosophy (and Theology) of Medicine

Introduction

A key assumption in much bioethical discussion is that bioethics can go along fairly well with minimal ontological and ethical commitments. For instance, Beauchamp and Childress apply a 'thin' proceduralist principlism to medical ethics, largely on the grounds that it's easier to agree on what we should do than on why we should do it.[1] Similarly, public discourse generally proceeds along the lines of a 'lowest common denominator ethics', which reduces (term used advisedly) ethical analysis to utilitarian calculus.[2] This is, in part, because its proponents believe that consideration of the *interests* of those affected by a decision or policy makes no assumptions about the nature of those interests, nor does it entail commitment to an underlying set of beliefs or values that would be controversial in the marketplace of ideas. I would contend that such approaches arise out of 'modernist' commitments to such things as a consensus view of (moral) reasoning and the distinction between a public realm of 'facts' and a private realm of 'values'; but let me leave that to one side for the moment.

1 Tom L. Beauchamp, The 'Four Principles' Approach, in *Meaning and Medicine: A Reader in the Philosophy of Health Care*, ed. J. L. Nelson and H. L. Nelson (New York: Routledge, 1999); cf. the critique in K. Danner Clouser and Bernard Gert, A Critique of Principlism, in *Meaning and Medicine: A Reader in the Philosophy of Health Care*, ed. J. L. Nelson and H. L. Nelson (New York: Routledge, 1999).

2 So, for instance, despite the importance of other lines of argument, *reporting* of the case for and against the creation of 'three-parent embryos' focused almost exclusively on the consequences of the policy. See, for instance, http://www.telegraph.co.uk/news/science/science-news/11386151/Three-parent-babies-the-arguments-for-and-against.html (accessed 13/03/2015).

In bioethics, then, the idea seems to be that we can proceed to concrete decision-making without a clearly identified moral or philosophical rationale. It is my contention that (a) this is not possible; (b) it results in substantive ontological and moral questions being hidden rather than excluded from decision-making; (c) it fails to address key aspects of the world that should be analysed (including the nature of medicine itself); (d) it leaves unchallenged basic assumptions that need to be brought to light and subjected to critical appraisal.[3]

These are big claims, which have serious implications for our understanding and practice of bioethics. I will seek to demonstrate them in relation to two issues, one deeply contested and clearly problematic, the other apparently more straightforward. I will look first at euthanasia (or assisted dying), an obvious contender given its prominence in public discussions and the intractable nature of the debates surrounding it. I will identify and analyse the main arguments used to support the case 'for' and the case 'against' euthanasia, using an exemplar of each case for the sake of clarity. In doing so, I aim to show that along with issues such as the nature of autonomy and of human dignity, deeper questions relating to the nature and goals of medicine fuel the debate. I will then turn to the ethics of organ transplantation. Rather than canvas a range of views on transplantation *per se* (for there is general agreement that organ transplantation is a 'good thing'), I will focus on Janet Radcliffe Richards' arguments for why we need to change public policies and attitudes in order to increase the 'supply' of organs for donation.[4] I'll begin by briefly outlining her case for her central claims, before seeking to identify the (unstated) ethical theory that drives it. I'll then move on to explore some of the underlying philosophical issues relating to the nature of persons and of medicine that

[3] These claims are echoed by a number of authors in relation to a number of issues. See, for instance, James M. Gustafson, Theology Confronts Technology and the Life Sciences, *Commonweal* 105 (1978); H. Tristram Engelhardt, Jr, Bioethics at the End of the Millennium: Fashioning Health Care Policy in the Absence of a Moral Consensus, in *Ethical Issues in Health Care on the Frontiers of the Twenty-First Century*, ed. Stephen Wear et al. (Dordrecht: Kluwer, 2000); Christian Bioethics after Christendom: Living in a Secular Fundamentalist Polity and Culture, *Christian Bioethics: Non-Ecumenical Studies in Medical Morality* 17, no. 1 (2011); Global Bioethics, Theology, and Human Genetic Engineering: The Challenge of Refashioning Human Nature in the Face of Moral and Religious Pluralism, in *GenEthics and Religion*, ed. G. Phleiderer, G. Brahier, and K. Lindpaintner (Basel: Krager, 2010); Lisa Sowle Cahill, Theologians and Bioethicists: Some History and a Proposal, in *On Moral Medicine: Theological Perspectives in Medical Ethics*, ed. M. Therese Lysaught et al. (Grand Rapids: Eerdmans, 2012).

[4] Janet Radcliffe Richards, *The Ethics of Transplants: Why Careless Thought Costs Lives* (Oxford: Oxford University Press, 2012).

inform her case, before suggesting that this kind of analysis can and should be brought to bear on other (I would argue all) discussions in bioethics, the ethics of medicine and related matters.

Euthanasia

Setting the scene: debates about assisted dying in the Western world

Few issues have the prominence in discussions of medical ethics and bioethics in either the public sphere or the academy that abortion and euthanasia have been given. And even fewer are more controversial and none, perhaps, generate such strong feelings as do these touchstone issues. Here, I will focus on euthanasia, in part because it is a more 'live' issue (so to speak) in general political discourse than abortion, largely due to the currency of debates on the legalizing of 'assisted dying' in a number of jurisdictions.[5] I will briefly outline the main arguments for and against the practice of euthanasia, paying particular attention to Peter Singer's case for it and John Wyatt's case against it. I will then seek to identify the underlying ethical perspectives that inform their cases and the philosophical (and theological) commitments entailed in them.[6] My aim,

5 When I began writing this chapter, Lord Falconer of Thoroton's Private Members' Bill had received its first reading in the UK House of Lords (http://services.parliament.uk/bills/2013-14/assisteddying.html; accessed 05/03/2014); the Australian Green party's policies include legalizing voluntary euthanasia (http://greens.org.au/dying-with-dignity; accessed 05/03/2014); while US federal law prohibits euthanasia, the US states of Oregon, Vermont and Washington have legalized physician-assisted suicide, while in Montana physician-assisted suicide is legal as a result of a court ruling (http://euthanasia.procon.org/view.resource.php?resourceID=000132; accessed 05/03/2014); in Europe, while France is considering legalizing euthanasia, both euthanasia and physician-assisted suicide are legal in Belgium, the Netherlands and Luxembourg, and physician-assisted suicide is legal in Switzerland (http://euthanasia.procon.org/view.resource.php?resourceID=000136; accessed 05/03/2014).

6 While it makes obvious sense to speak of John Wyatt's theological commitments – given that he explicitly identifies himself as an evangelical Christian and outlines a theological framework for the issues he addresses (see John Wyatt, *Matters of Life and Death: Human Dilemmas in the Light of the Christian Faith* (Nottingham: IVP, 2009), 15–24), it may seem odd to speak of Peter Singer's theological commitments given that he explicitly identifies himself as an atheist and outlines arguments against key theological propositions (see, for instance, Peter Singer, *Rethinking Life and Death* (Melbourne: Text, 1994), esp. 1–5, 187–222). However, following Alvin Plantinga's lead (in Alvin Plantinga, *God, Freedom and Evil* (New York: Harper and Row, 1974)), we can speak meaningfully of the metaphysical assumptions that lie in the conceptual background of atheism and see them as articulating an a-theological line, hence engaging in a kind of theology (even if a theology of radical denial).

however, is not to attempt to adjudicate between the arguments, but to demonstrate that debates in bioethics hinge on underlying substantive issues, including a basic understanding of medicine and what it is for, and so show that bioethics demonstrates the value of and need for philosophy and theology of medicine. I will return to these issues later, to see what light is shed on the debate by philosophical and theological reflection on the nature and goals of medicine.[7]

The 'pro-choice' case for assisted dying

Many lines of argument have been used to justify the practice of euthanasia and its legalization. The most common one, and that which seems to me to be most central to the arguments in favour of euthanasia, is that of individual autonomy. Simply put, the principle of respect for autonomy states that each individual has the right to conduct their own affairs and make whichever choices they see fit, so long as this does not impinge on another person's exercise of their own rights. This basic principle, it is argued, entails a right to die: for any limitation of my decision to end my life is an imposition of another person's will on my right to determine the manner and timing of my death. The existence of such a right, it is claimed, is an implication of the value and inherent dignity of human (or self-aware) life.

There are a number of important supporting arguments in the case for euthanasia. There is no relevant ethical distinction between killing (euthanasia) and letting die (withdrawal of therapy and provision of palliative care): death is the end in each case, there is no relevant difference in the nature of the acts themselves, and death is envisaged, or even willed, as the end in both cases; thus, they are equivalent ethically. Euthanasia is compassionate: suffering is only tolerable if it is in the service of a greater good; for terminally ill people, there is no such good; thus, suffering should be terminated, by death if necessary.[8] Voluntary euthanasia upholds the importance of *quality* of life

[7] See Chapter 9.

[8] It is interesting to note the way this upholds McKenny's claim that modern medicine, and the bioethics associated with it, sees suffering as inherently meaningless, for which see Gerald P. McKenny, *To Relieve the Human Condition: Bioethics, Technology, and the Body* (Albany: University of New York Press, 1997), esp. 211–226.

versus its mere continuance. The benefits of euthanasia outweigh its drawbacks: it will alleviate suffering, promote autonomy, save the community wasted resources, and allay the fears of many elderly and dying people that their deaths will be undignified and attended by pointless suffering.[9]

The 'pro-life' case against assisted dying

A similar range of arguments has been used to oppose the institution of voluntary euthanasia. The main traditional argument against euthanasia is the doctrine of the sanctity of (human) life. Human beings are seen as distinct from all other creatures, with unique inherent value which euthanasia violates. In Judaeo-Christian thought, this is usually seen as a derivative of humanity's being created uniquely in the image of God. The argument is as follows. Life is God's gift, and it is his prerogative alone to give or withhold it. To deliberately take my own life, or that of another innocent human being, it is argued, is to despise God's gift, and violate the sanctity of human life. An important supporting argument is that there is a relevant distinction between euthanasia and the withdrawal or withholding of life-prolonging therapy, which means that the latter is justified in some circumstances, even though the person's life may be shortened as a result, whereas the former is not. This is usually based on one or more of three grounds: the distinction between killing and letting die; the doctrine of double effect; or the difference between the ethical status of 'ordinary' ('proportionate') versus 'extraordinary' ('disproportionate') therapy.

There are a number of supplementary arguments cited against the practice of voluntary euthanasia. There are crucial philosophical and theological problems with the particular notion of autonomy used to justify euthanasia: we are not autonomous in that sense, and so autonomy is either irrelevant to

[9] For presentations of some or all of these arguments, see: Paul Badham, Should Christians Accept the Validity of Voluntary Euthanasia?, *Studies in Christian Ethics* 8, no. 2 (1995); Tony Delamothe, Rosamund Snow, and Fiona Godlee, Why the Assisted Dying Bill Should Become Law in England and Wales, *British Medical Journal* 349 (2014); Gerald Dworkin, Physician-Assisted Death: The State of the Debate, in *The Oxford Handbook of Bioethics*, ed. Bonnie Steinbock (Oxford: Oxford University Press, 2007); Hans Kung, A Dignified Dying, in *On Moral Medicine: Theological Perspectives in Medical Ethics*, ed. M. Therese Lysaught et al. (Grand Rapids: Eerdmans, 2012); James Rachels, Active and Passive Euthanasia, in *Killing and Letting Die*, ed. Bonnie Steinbock (Englewood Cliffs: Prentice Hall, 1980); Michael Tooley, An Irrelevant Consideration: Killing versus Letting Die, in *Killing and Letting Die*, ed. Bonnie Steinbock (Englewood Cliffs: Prentice Hall, 1980).

the debate or (when properly understood) works against legalizing euthanasia. True compassion entails care for the dying, not their death. Euthanasia conflicts with the essence, or central features, of the practice of medicine. Legalizing euthanasia would have many unacceptable consequences: it would distort the nature and practice of medicine; it would undermine the traditional doctor–patient relationship; there is the danger of the 'slippery slope' – voluntary euthanasia could lead to non-voluntary, or even involuntary, euthanasia; it will become an easy way out for patients and society, resulting in problems with the allocation of adequate resources to palliative care services; it runs the risk of misplaced and coerced altruism – the elderly or infirm believing or being 'told' that they have a 'duty to die' so as not to be a burden to others or society.[10]

Peter Singer on euthanasia

Turning to the analysis of the cases for and against euthanasia and the way they indicate the need for a philosophy (and theology) of medicine, I will first examine Peter Singer's case for euthanasia. In Chapter 1 of *Practical Ethics*, 'About Ethics', Singer outlines his ethical theory, namely *preference utilitarianism*, and briefly justifies that view *vis-à-vis* some of its main rivals.[11] He is clear in avowing that this comprises more an outline of 'the assumptions on which the rest of the book is based', than a defence of them.[12] He argues that we ought to govern our ethical decisions on the basis of the (predicted) consequences of

10 For presentations of some or all of these arguments, see D. J. Atkinson, Causing Death and Allowing to Die, *Tyndale Bulletin* 34 (1983); Dietrich Bonhoeffer, *Ethics*, trans. N. H. Smith (London: SCM, 1955), 131–147; James F. Keenan, The Case for Physician-Assisted Suicide?, in *On Moral Medicine: Theological Perspectives in Medical Ethics*, ed. M. Therese Lysaught et al. (Grand Rapids: Eerdmans, 2012); N. Lickiss, Euthanasia from the Perspective of a Palliative Care Consultant (paper presented at the Proceedings of Conference on Active Voluntary Euthanasia, Monash University Centre for Human Bioethics, 15/11/1993); Gordon Preece, Rethinking Singer on Life and Death, in *Rethinking Peter Singer: A Christian Critique*, ed. Gordon Preece (Downers Grove: IVP, 2002); Gilbert Meilaender, *Bioethics: A Primer for Christians*, 3rd edn. (Grand Rapids: Eerdmans, 2013), 57–78; J. P. Moreland, James Rachels and the Active Euthanasia Debate, *Journal of the Evangelical Theological Society* 31, no. 1 (1988); Paul Ramsey, *Ethics at the Edges of Life: Medical and Legal Intersections* (New Haven: Yale University Press, 1978), 145–188. See also my discussion of Pope John Paul II and Nigel M. de S. Cameron in Chapter 5.

11 Peter Singer, *Practical Ethics*, 2nd edn. (Cambridge: Cambridge University Press, 1993), 1–15 [*Practical Ethics*, 3rd edn. (Cambridge: Cambridge University Press, 2009), 1–15]. From here on, I will cite the references to the 3rd edition in square brackets where they differ from those of the 2nd edition.

12 *Practical Ethics*, 1, 8, 14–15.

how measured ?

our actions, considering *all* who are likely to be affected by that decision, not just ourselves.[13] More specifically, we should choose whichever line of action has 'the best consequences', where desirable consequences are understood as those which 'further the interests' of those affected by a given decision.[14] At the close of that chapter, he states: 'I am inclined to hold a utilitarian position, and to some extent the book may be taken as an attempt to indicate how a consistent utilitarianism would deal with a number of controversial problems.'[15]

In Chapter 7, 'Taking Life: Humans', in which he deals with the ethics of taking human life, Singer applies his earlier arguments to euthanasia. In so doing, he rehearses many of the arguments I mentioned above: autonomy and human dignity, in favour of voluntary euthanasia, and against involuntary euthanasia;[16] beneficial consequences for the person, in favour of voluntary and non-voluntary euthanasia and infanticide;[17] beneficial consequences for the parents or others in favour of infanticide.[18] Now, it is not my purpose to detail those arguments or their refutation, because, while I believe these arguments can be refuted,[19] that lies beyond my scope here, which is to demonstrate that Singer's arguments and conclusions on euthanasia are an expression of his general ethical theory, and depend upon it for their justification. This is clearly the case in his positive arguments for euthanasia, as he repeatedly refers to preference utilitarianism as the rationale for his adopting a particular argument or conclusion.[20] It is equally clear in his refutation of arguments against euthanasia. For instance, he claims a number of times that the 'sanctity of life principle' has been refuted. Indeed, he goes so far as to claim that 'the doctrines about sanctity of human life' 'collapse as soon as they are questioned'.[21] Whether that is the case or not, when his arguments against the

13 *Practical Ethics*, 8–14.
14 *Practical Ethics*, 13–14.
15 *Practical Ethics*, 14–15 [14]. He goes on to say that he attempts to show how other viewpoints bear upon the issues. However, this attempt is often cursory, even contemptuous, at least in the case of deontological perspectives, especially those which hold to versions of the 'sanctity of (human) life principle', as can be seen on p.175 [155].
16 *Practical Ethics*, 193–196, 199–201 [169–171, 175–177].
17 *Practical Ethics*, 183–193 [161–169].
18 *Practical Ethics*, 182–183, 185–188 [160–161, 162–165].
19 For this, see Preece, Rethinking Peter Singer.
20 Singer, *Practical Ethics*, 181–201 [159–178].
21 *Practical Ethics*, 175 [155].

principle are reviewed, they all are based upon his preference utilitarian stance.[22] His arguments against specific counters to a pro-euthanasia stance are equally reliant on his preference utilitarianism.[23] While there are epistemological flaws in appraising a theory or intellectual tradition solely from a perspective external to it, this clearly demonstrates his reliance upon his theoretical perspective in case of specific arguments for his view and against its rivals.

I believe, however, that this can be taken further. Not only do his views on specific issues reflect his global theory of ethics, but his ethical theory is an articulation of his 'worldview', his fundamental understanding of the nature of reality and of humanity's place in it. This is seen in a number of ways. First, his adoption of preference utilitarianism and the specific views it gives rise to is in self-conscious opposition to what he calls the 'crumbling moral framework' of traditional ethics, in particular the Judaeo-Christian tradition.[24] Second, he specifically argues that this crumbling framework should be replaced by another, which arises out of a rival metaphysical vision.[25] Third, the very issues he addresses in his book reflect a hierarchy of values which arises out of a particular worldview.[26] Finally, in Chapter 12 of *Practical Ethics*, 'Why Act Morally?', he looks at the question of the philosophical (meta-ethical) justification of the moral point of view.[27] This justification, he argues, depends upon a particular understanding of human nature, purpose and our interaction with the universe in which the ethical point of view *itself* provides the person-transcendent meaning and purpose which older worldviews found in theism. This (quasi) metaphysical position justifies his adoption of the ethical point of view, and indeed the kind of ethical theory he adopts.[28] I think this demonstrates that stances on euthanasia, ethical vision and worldview are deeply entangled in Peter Singer's case.

[22] See *Practical Ethics*, Ch. 4, What's Wrong with Killing?, where he establishes the grounds for his 'anti-speciesist' stance on equality of consideration for humans and animals.

[23] *Practical Ethics*, 202–217 [178–190].

[24] *Practical Ethics*, 3–4, 83–89 [3–4, 71–76]; *Rethinking Life and Death*, esp. 1–6, 159–183, 187–222.

[25] *Rethinking Life and Death*, 187–222.

[26] *Practical Ethics*, 1–2. For instance, he considers the ethics of sex to be relatively unproblematic and unimportant in comparison with the environment or international justice. This may be true, but clearly reflects a hierarchical valuation arising out of a broader view of life.

[27] *Practical Ethics*, 314–335 [276–295].

[28] *Practical Ethics*, 331–335 [291–295].

More can be made, however, of the link between the case for euthanasia and the view of medicine and human community that informs it. As noted earlier, at the centre of the case for euthanasia is the notion of autonomy, understood in a particular way. Autonomy is seen as the freedom for an individual to make decisions about themselves and their future without reference to anything other than their will, so long as this does not impinge on another's freedom to do the same. This fits with late capitalism's commitment to consumer choice and the libertarian ideals that go along with it. This libertarian view of autonomy reflects a basic understanding of human personhood and the nature of human community. Notions of transcendent values or an ultimate *telos* of human existence no longer ground our understanding of the nature and purpose of humanity. Whereas in the past, it is claimed, ethics was governed by notions of a transcendent god or gods whose will was expressed in a moral law, or of an ultimate goal that controlled our understanding of human nature and purpose,[29] these metaphysical claims are otiose, being either unwarranted or unnecessary. In their absence, we are able to value human beings as those who are able to govern their own existence, creating meaning and value for themselves by way of the enterprises they adopt and into which they invest themselves. Without a transcendent grounding of the 'human project', we are able to determine the nature of our own life project, and must be free to do so without the constraints of outdated social values that are illegitimate impositions of outmoded and minority religious views. Others are entitled to adopt those views if they wish; they are not entitled to foist them on others by way of legal restrictions on the freely made decisions of others. The end is the kind of libertarian autonomy championed by proponents of euthanasia.

Medicine, then, as a social institution, has value in as much as it enables people to overcome the limitations of the human condition and enact their freely made decisions and navigate the world as agents.[30] Those decisions, in order to be free, must be properly informed; nonetheless, there are no other legitimate restrictions on those decisions except those that are necessary in

29 These giving morality some transcendent grounding of one kind or another: either by some connection with the divine will (be that expressed in terms of commandments or principles, or the ultimate ends of human existence of Thomistic natural law ethics); or as a way of grasping 'moral facts' (such as Kantian categorical imperatives, or Platonic ideals, or Aristotelian natural law).

30 McKenny, *To Relieve the Human Condition*, esp. Chapters 1 and 2.

order to grant others the same freedom. Illness, infirmity and suffering impinge on our freedom, and so ought to be combatted, and medicine is an efficient way of doing so. It has, however, no more moral freight than that which its role as an enabler of human autonomy can bear. If legalizing euthanasia changes the way we see medicine, health care and their associated practices, then this is not a *distortion* of medicine, but an expression of its nature and purpose, perhaps an unveiling of its true nature and purpose once we strip away the unreasonable and restrictive views of those who claim otherwise. I will say more about these issues later, but for now I think my point is clear: the arguments for euthanasia articulate deeper ethical theories and philosophical commitments, including underlying concepts of the nature and goals of medicine. This shows that examining such concepts has instrumental value (given that it will help us understand better such intractable debates), as well as suggesting that it has intrinsic value (given the importance of medicine in contemporary societies).

John Wyatt on euthanasia

John Wyatt is equally explicit that his arguments against euthanasia arise out of his underlying Christian theological and ethical views, as the subtitle of his book makes clear.[31] Having presented a description of the current state of the art of medicine and biotechnology,[32] he explicitly outlines a Christian 'worldview', focusing on its implications for our understanding of humanity.[33] He outlines a broadly 'redemptive-history' framework of creation, fall, redemption and consummation, focusing on what it implies or entails concerning our understanding of human existence as individuals and in community. While no one can do everything, it is interesting that he explicates neither the shape of his overarching ethical theory nor a more comprehensive view of medicine,[34]

[31] Wyatt, *Matters of Life and Death*, subtitled: *Human Dilemmas in the Light of the Christian Faith.*

[32] *Matters of Life and Death*, 25–49.

[33] *Matters of Life and Death*, 51–82.

[34] To be fair, he does address some of those issues in Chapters 1 and 11, but the discussion in Chapter 11 can clearly play no structural role in his earlier analysis (as it comes so late in the book), and that of Chapter 1 plays only an introductory role and is not explicitly brought to bear on his analysis of cases and issues (see *Matters of Life and Death*, 25–49, 239–263). I will argue below, however, that an implicit ethical theory and understanding of medicine and its role in human community does inform his analysis.

presuming that a 'sanctity of life' ethic is adequate to ground his subsequent discussion. However, it seems clear that his is a broadly deontological (and absolutist) approach to ethics in which the sanctity or dignity of human life as creatures made in God's image gives rise to principles that control how we should understand and treat each other.[35] While he doesn't expound the (meta-ethical) nature of his ethics, Wyatt is explicit that his understanding of Christian faith controls his conclusions on the matters at hand. In this respect, he, like Singer, seeks to bring his general ethical views to bear on particular ethical concerns.

In Chapter 9, 'A Good Death? Euthanasia and Assisted Suicide', he outlines the context and reasons behind the move towards legalizing euthanasia,[36] before turning to his own views in Chapter 10, 'A Better Way to Die'.[37] Wyatt utilizes a number of the typical anti-euthanasia arguments I outlined earlier. As I've already noted, Wyatt's chief argument against euthanasia and for the provision of appropriate (palliative) care for the dying is that euthanasia conflicts with a commitment to human dignity and the sanctity of human life as grounded in our being made in God's image. He is equally clear in his avowal of a distinction between killing and letting die, in part due to his refusal to allow ethical analysis to be reduced to the appraisal of the consequences of our actions or policies, but also because of his acceptance of the doctrine of double effect and of the difference between ordinary care and extraordinary care.[38] Similarly, he puts forward most of the typical ancillary arguments against euthanasia. I should note in passing that much of his discussion in Chapter 9 (where most of these counter-arguments are found) mixes description and ethical analysis somewhat indiscriminately,[39] and he uses fear as a governing category, which I'm not convinced is quite right.[40] Nonetheless, he endorses the main ancillary arguments, and in pretty much their usual form: the notion of

35 See, for instance, *Matters of Life and Death*, 56, 60–63, 78–79, 158–162. This is, of course, in contrast to many traditional Roman Catholic approaches which, while similarly absolutist, articulate a sanctity of life ethic in terms of teleology and natural law (see, for instance, Pope John Paul II, *Evangelium Vitae* (Rome: Vatican, 1995)).

36 Wyatt, *Matters of Life and Death*, 191–214.

37 *Matters of Life and Death*, 215–237.

38 *Matters of Life and Death*, 215–237.

39 *Matters of Life and Death*, esp. 192, 194–197, 200–204, 212–214.

40 *Matters of Life and Death*, 197–200.

autonomy that justifies euthanasia is flawed;[41] compassion entails care for the dying, not their death;[42] euthanasia conflicts with the tradition of Hippocratic medicine;[43] legalizing euthanasia would have many unacceptable consequences, including the risk of the law being abused;[44] both the arguments for and practice of voluntary euthanasia starts us on a slippery slope which may lead to involuntary euthanasia and euthanasia on grounds other than terminal illness or great suffering;[45] it will become an easy solution to problems of resource allocation, further exacerbating the pressures on care for the elderly, disabled and dying, and risking their neglect;[46] it runs the risk of misplaced and coerced altruism.[47]

Once again, my purpose here is not to appraise the relative strengths and weaknesses of his arguments, but to show how they both articulate his underlying ethical stance and imply a particular vision of human life in community and of medicine within it. It is clear that his sanctity of life ethic governs his arguments. Life is God's gift, and it is God's prerogative to determine its end; for us to take a human being's life, even out of (misguided) compassion, is to despise the giver of the gift and fail to respect human dignity. Furthermore, medicine does not exist to overcome the exigencies of creaturely finitude, but to reverse the effects of the brokenness of creation and of human sin and to care for people in the midst of it, thereby demonstrating a commitment to them as creatures with inherent dignity.

Wyatt draws a crucial distinction that exemplifies his understanding of both medicine and its limits. Using the analogy of an artwork, he sees medicine's role as *restorative*, not *creative* or *constructive*.[48] That is, medicine is in the business of correcting what's gone wrong, be that by way of congenital abnormality, disease process, injury or disability, not in the business of

[41] *Matters of Life and Death*, 199–200, 219–220, 231.
[42] *Matters of Life and Death*, 229–233. He adds that it wrongly buys into the notion that suffering is ultimately meaningless, and robs people of the difficult gift of dying well (pp. 219–220, 226–229).
[43] *Matters of Life and Death*, 194–195, 207–208, 239–263. The question of just how important the prohibition of euthanasia is in the Hippocratic tradition is a disputed question; but adjudicating that claim is not relevant to my argument at this point.
[44] *Matters of Life and Death*, 202, 205–214, 233–234.
[45] *Matters of Life and Death*, 202–205.
[46] *Matters of Life and Death*, 202, 212–214.
[47] *Matters of Life and Death*, 201.
[48] *Matters of Life and Death*, 99–100.

enhancement. Furthermore, medicine needs to accept the limits God has established, limits that arise both from the inherent dignity of being those created in the image of God and from creaturely finitude. Thus, any medical 'treatment' that transgresses against human dignity is illegitimate; so too is any that struggles against the inevitable weaknesses and dependencies of human mortality. In as much as euthanasia fails to respect human dignity and seeks mastery over mortality (and the fears associated with it in a culture constructed around notions of individualistic autonomy), it conflicts with the *ethos* of medicine and so cannot be justified from a Christian point of view.

I do not claim that these reflections are radical or novel or new; nor (at this stage) will I seek to adjudicate between the arguments for and against euthanasia. My aim here is simply to show that without discussing those deeper philosophical (and theological) issues relating to the nature of humanity and human existence, human community and the goods and goals proper to it, and the nature and role of medicine in light of our broader social agenda, we cannot adequately discuss the issues. Of course, this may not lead to any kind of consensus on the matters; it may not even allow for the identifying of common ground on which we can hammer out some kind of consensus. I do not claim that this analysis can help *resolve* intractable debates, simply that it might help us better understand why they are so intractable and gain clarity as to where the arguments ought to be directed (not, I would suggest, at the detail of specific arguments about the logic of distinctions between killing and letting die, for instance, but at the underlying views of humanity, community and medicine that inform them).[49]

Now, it may be thought that in choosing to examine arguments for and against euthanasia, I have given myself too easy a task: in a matter such as this, it is obvious that ethical arguments relate to broader philosophical and theological commitments and so easy to make a case for bioethics needing a philosophy (and theology) of medicine. It is clear, even from my brief discussion of a couple of representative exponents, that much of the argument

[49] For a helpful discussion of the arguments, and their impact (or lack thereof) on medical practice, which also notes the importance of underlying concepts of medicine in this debate, see Denise Anne Cooper, The Doctor as Moral Agent, with Reference to the Distinction between Killing and 'Letting Die' (PhD, The University of Melbourne, 2007).

hinges on the cogency or otherwise of arguments for or against human dignity or the sanctity of human life and their implications, positions adopted on the nature and limitations of autonomy, and so on. And it is fairly apparent that deeper metaphysical and a/theological views underpin those arguments and viewpoints. This is explicitly the case with Papal declarations and Wyatt's opposition to euthanasia. It is less explicit but equally apparent in Singer's advocacy of it. Debates over such an intractable issue, like the question of abortion with which it is often connected, might be expected to have their roots in conflicting 'worldviews'. So, let me turn to another issue entirely, one concerning a much less controversial matter: organ transplantation, a practice that has received support from a broad cross-section of people, ranging from the Vatican to Peter Singer.

Janet Radcliffe Richards on organ transplantation

Organ transplantation has been one of the many success stories of modern, high-tech medicine. Since the first kidney transplant in 1950, both the range of organs that can be successfully transplanted and transplant success has boomed. In 2014, there were 1,193 organ transplants in Australia;[50] 4,655 in the UK;[51] 29,533 in the US.[52] Globally, there were around 100,800 solid organ transplants in 2008.[53] Transplant surgery has, however, become something of a victim of its own success: one of the major restrictions on the provision of transplant services is the availability of organs for transplantation. These restrictions are both practical and moral: there is a limit on the availability of solid organs for transplant (especially vital non-paired organs such as the heart, since the donor cannot survive the donation); and there are limitations on the circumstances in which donation can rightly be made. So, despite the

50 This included 659 kidney, 237 liver, 79 heart, 4 heart/lung, 159 lung and 54 pancreas transplants; http://www.donatelife.gov.au/discover/facts-and-statistics (accessed 13/03/2015).

51 This included 3,257 kidney, 924 liver, 206 heart, 218 lung, 261 pancreas and 26 bowel transplants; http://www.organdonation.nhs.uk/statistics/ (accessed 13/03/2015).

52 This included 17,107 kidney, 6,729 liver, 2,655 heart, 1,925 lung, 709 kidney/pancreas, 245 pancreas, 139 bowel and 24 heart/lung transplants; http://optn.transplant.hrsa.gov/ (accessed 13/03/2015).

53 This included 69,400 kidney, 20,200 liver, 5,400 heart, 3,400 lung and 2,400 pancreas transplants; http://www.who.int/transplantation/gkt/statistics/en/ (accessed 13/03/2015).

dramatic increase in successful transplant surgery, there are around 1,500 people on the waiting list for organs in Australia;[54] 7,000 in the UK;[55] 123,000 in the US;[56] and the worldwide waiting list for a kidney for transplant alone exceeds 200,000.[57] These are the issues that Janet Radcliffe Richards addresses, as is fairly obvious from the title of her book, *The Ethics of Transplants*. What is also obvious (from the subtitle, *Why Careless Thought Costs Lives*) is the line that she pursues in the book.[58] Her argument is that there are many unnecessary barriers placed on the procurement of organs for transplant due to faulty moral reasoning.

Radcliffe Richards makes clear her starting point and governing idea in her introductory chapter: 'I shall take as a starting proposition the claim that if someone's life or health can be saved by means of a transplant, that is in itself a good thing . . . It follows from this that if someone is dying or ill, and could be saved for a life worth living by a transplant, there is a *presumption* in favour of bringing that about whenever possible.'[59] Furthermore, in light of limited availability of organs for transplants, there is a corresponding 'presumption in favour of any policy that opens up a potential source of organs, and conversely against any policy that closes or curtails one'.[60] Now, these are *prima facie* judgements, not conclusions made all-things-considered; nonetheless, those presumptions guide the argument of the rest of the book, both in content and in tone.

Chapter 2, 'Procurement from the Living', seeks to overcome one of the chief impediments to procuring organs, particularly kidneys, from living people: namely, the ban on payment. Her argument focuses on how we ought to construe our rights to our organs, concluding that it makes best sense to view them as a version of property rights. This then means that people ought to be free to make informed decisions about how they dispose of this property,

54 http://www.donatelife.gov.au/discover/facts-and-statistics (accessed 13/03/2015).

55 https://nhsbtmediaservices.blob.core.windows.net/organ-donation-assets/pdfs/annual_stats.pdf (accessed 13/03/2015).

56 http://optn.transplant.hrsa.gov/ (accessed 13/03/2015).

57 http://www.who.int/bulletin/volumes/85/1/07-020107/en/ (accessed 13/03/2015).

58 It is interesting to note that in the paperback edition of her book, title and subtitle are reversed: *Careless Thought Costs Lives: The Ethics of Transplants* (Oxford: Oxford University Press, 2013).

59 Radcliffe Richards, *The Ethics of Transplants*, 14–15.

60 *The Ethics of Transplants*, 16.

including, for instance, selling a kidney for a significant sum. She identifies what she sees as the impediments to such a policy and systematically counters them. Chapter 3, 'Methodological Morals', outlines what she sees as the form of sound moral arguments and both the reasons for and significance of the failure of arguments against paid organ procurement. She presents her analysis as neutral and objective, entailing no substantive moral commitments (other than being in favour of maximizing organ transplantation). Chapter 4, 'Procurement from the Dead', outlines an argument along similar lines to that of Chapter 2 in favour of people being able, within practical limits, to 'will' their organs rather than them being impartially allocated, as well as suggesting that only those who are willing to 'donate' organs ought to be able to receive one should the need arise. The final chapter, 'Penumbral Problems', deals largely with questions relating to the 'dead donor rule' and procuring organs from those who are 'brain dead' (or in related conditions in the shadowy borderlands between life and death). She notes the now familiar problems with notions such as 'brain death' as a determinant of the death of a person and outlines the equally familiar solution of disposing of the 'dead donor rule' and allowing for organs to be procured from those who can no longer benefit from them in order to benefit those who can. Her conclusion is clear, and predictable from both the nature of her arguments and the subtitle of her book: careless thought in all these areas – especially thought encumbered by the shibboleths of traditional moral intuitions – illegitimately restricts the availability of organs for transplantation and so costs lives.

Digging deeper

Underlying ethical theory

So, how does Radcliffe Richards' case demonstrate bioethics' need for a philosophy and theology of medicine? That requires digging a little deeper and seeking to expose the underlying lineaments of her case. The first step is to identify the ethical theory that undergirds her argument, before proceeding to bring to light the unstated assumptions about the nature of human beings, community and the nature and goals of medicine that inform her discussion.

I will begin by analysing her ethical framework, doing so by picking out an early section of argument, before showing how this is exemplified in the rest of the book.

Early in the book, she discusses a somewhat *outré* thought experiment of John Harris: the suggestion that we should introduce a 'survival lottery'. The idea is this:

> Whenever half a dozen people needing transplants could be saved by the organs of a single person, lots would be drawn to see which healthy individual should be sacrificed to save the six in need. The chances of anyone's being drawn in the lottery would be far lower than that of their dying prematurely from organ failure at some point in their lives. Interestingly, however, it seems that nobody confronted with this thought experiment would choose to join any such scheme.[61]

Having outlined the case for it, and given some thought as to why people would rationally resist it, she presents the following argument against our adopting it:

> It is intrinsically good to save lives.
>
> If we had enough organs, transplantation could save many more lives than it currently does.
>
> We could save all these lives, and increase everyone's statistical life expectancy, if we instituted some kind of survival lottery.
>
> *But . . . It seems to be a deep fact about human nature that we regard many things as more important than life expectancy, and, even with full understanding and after careful consideration, few people would be willing to purchase additional life expectancy at the cost of entering a survival lottery.*
>
> *We should not put in place arrangements that would please nobody.*
>
> -------------------
>
> Therefore we should *not* institute a survival lottery.[62]

To understand what theory informs this argument, it is worth noting which considerations are excluded or ignored in her argument, and which are factored in. There are a number of obvious exclusions, largely relating to questions of the nature of the action and of the kinds of persons and institutions

[61] *The Ethics of Transplants*, 18.
[62] *The Ethics of Transplants*, 21.

that might enact such a programme. These are, broadly speaking, the focus of deontological and virtue ethics. It is worth noticing, for instance, that she gives no consideration to the question of the character of a person who might be able to kill an innocent person for the benefit of others, or to the way in which participation in such practices might morally mal/form them. She also gives no thought to the institutional frameworks that would need to govern the practice. Questions of individual and institutional virtue or vice have no bearing on her appraisal of this thought experiment.

Equally, she pays no attention to whether killing an innocent person is intrinsically right or wrong, nor to the issue of whether that question is informed by notions of the inherent dignity or worth of a human being. That is evident, not only in the course of her argument, but in the fact that she engages in it: for no one who believed in the inherent dignity of the human person or the intrinsic wrongness of killing a human being is likely to even entertain this thought experiment. The very fact that it is imaginable indicates that these deontological concerns do not enter her appraisal of the case. This oversight is not isolated to her appraisal of Harris's thought experiment, but is typical of her argument. For instance, the 'intrinsic good' of organ transplantation is determined on the basis of utilitarian calculus, not the inherent dignity of the recipient. And, in fact, questions of inherent dignity are not just ignored in her analysis, they are explicitly discounted as either vacuous or mere expression of unreasoned moral sentiment.

The suggestion that hers is a narrowly (and reductionist) utilitarian appraisal is reinforced when we note the considerations that are included in her argument. Her dismissal of the 'survival lottery' is based on observable human behaviour and the underlying motivations of those who would refuse to participate in the 'lottery', despite its utility. That is, her conclusions are based on her analysis of the interests, or preferences, of those affected by such a policy. The theory that drives her discussion is, I would suggest, a version of utilitarianism, one akin to the 'preference utilitarianism' espoused by Peter Singer. Her (preference) utilitarianism is evident not just in this opening section but throughout her argument.[63]

[63] *The Ethics of Transplants*, 45, 94–101 are two clear instances; but a utilitarian perspective is pervasive throughout the book.

Now, while I am not persuaded that utilitarianism gives us an adequate account of human morality, what concerns me here is the claim that bioethics can be done without addressing underlying theoretical concerns, as Radcliffe Richards herself does, claiming that her analysis of the arguments is objective and not driven by other commitments.[64] It only *proves* the claim false in Radcliffe Richards' own case, but it is certainly suggestive.

Implicit philosophical commitments

In fact, there are a number of deeper philosophical commitments evident in her work (if not openly acknowledged). The first is her rejection of notions of the inherent dignity or worth of human beings, as noted earlier. That is evident, I think, from the start of her argument. The intrinsic good of organ transplantation depends, not on the way it indicates our valuing of (vulnerable) persons, but on the utility of such procedures for furthering their interests.[65] It is also clear in her work on moral reasoning, where she rejects the notion of inherent rights or human dignity because they either can be reduced to ways of protecting human interests, or cannot be articulated in those terms and so are 'mysterious' or unwarranted emotional commitments rather than reasonable moral claims.[66] Thus, in rejecting the idea that the dead have rights, she states: 'The whole point of surrounding us, in life, with a circle of rights that other people cannot infringe without consent is to make certain things dependent on our will, and set them beyond the scope of what can be done to us by others.'[67] This, it seems to me, reflects what has been called the 'nihilistic will' of (late/post) modernity,[68] in which human value is reduced to or necessarily expressed in (almost) unfettered autonomy. While this is generally associated with reductionist physicalism, it generally comes with an ironic disparaging of the body and human bodily life. The body becomes reduced to a 'tool' or instrument of the transcendent human will, to be (re)crafted and

64 *The Ethics of Transplants*, 103, 105.
65 *The Ethics of Transplants*, 14–16.
66 *The Ethics of Transplants*, 29, 76–78, 110–114.
67 *The Ethics of Transplants*, 161.
68 David Bentley Hart, God or Nothingness, in *I Am the Lord Your God: Christian Reflections on the Ten Commandments*, ed. Carl E. Braaten and Christopher R. Seitz (Grand Rapids: Eerdmans, 2005).

used (and, in the end, disposed of) in whatever way is consistent with atomistic notions of the autonomous human will.[69] Important issues of philosophical and theological anthropology are at stake here, and need to be explicitly addressed.

The second is her uncritical adoption of the values and analytical categories of late modern capitalism. Having rejected notions of inherent value in favour of the idea that rights are a way of defending the interests of persons, she seeks to identify what kind of rights we might have to our bodies (and body parts). Her conclusion: *property rights*. That is to say, the way she understands our relationship to our bodies is that of ownership. Thus, someone is entitled to treat their paired organs (such as a kidney) as a commodity that can be sold to a willing (and presumably compatible) recipient.[70] Similarly, when thinking about the dead, she explicitly states that an undertaker selling the blood they drain from a corpse would be wrong in the same way as stealing (and selling) their wedding ring.[71] Her use of the 'neutral' language of 'source' and 'procurement' equally suggests a view of organs as commodities to be utilized beneficially, without reference to the deeply personal contexts in which they are 'procured' and then utilized.[72] This reflects a common move in recent thinking about health care, which reduces it to a commodity in the marketplace and doctors – and other health-care workers – to providers of a good or service who have no right to question the purposes for which their services are to be used. I will return to this issue later.

This relates to a third problem in her argument, and one that bedevils much bioethical discourse. She tends to exclude all the personal, relational and institutional factors that go into a 'thick description' of something like medicine. She states that her book 'does not go into any of the physiological details, or the practical arrangements and problems, or statistics about waiting lists and life expectancy after transplant'.[73] This is common in the literature (as evident, for

69 Jeffrey P. Bishop, *The Anticipatory Corpse: Medicine, Power and the Care of the Dying* (Notre Dame, IN: UNDP, 2011), esp. Chs 6–7; McKenny, *To Relieve the Human Condition*, esp. Chs 1–3, 7.

70 Radcliffe Richards, *The Ethics of Transplants*, Ch. 2. This coheres with my claim that the body is reduced to a tool of the autonomous will.

71 *The Ethics of Transplants*, 165.

72 *The Ethics of Transplants*, 2, 30.

73 *The Ethics of Transplants*, 27.

instance, in the classical essay by James Rachels,[74] in which he rejects the distinction between killing and letting die). However, it is precisely these practical arrangements, clinical contexts and personal features that give a complex social practice like medicine its character (pun intended). In order to understand what is going on in organ transplantation, we need to understand something of the procedures used, both in 'procuring' and in transplanting the organs; think about what they do to people, what they say about us and the relationships that are so crucial to, even constitutive of, human existence; how they relate to broader social expectations and aspirations and their connection to health care; and how they reflect (and shape) the nature of medicine.[75] The absence of such a 'thick description' is particularly striking in her discussion of people being able to 'will' their organs – that is to say, direct who might receive them after their death – where she simply ignores concerns ranging from histocompatibility to the relational implications of and institutional frameworks required for such a practice.[76]

Related to this is her failure to address a number of basic assumptions about organ transplantation and what it says about the nature and goal of medicine. She considers it as a treatment option like any other, the justification of which lies in its ability to forestall death or reduce suffering. That assumes, of course, that medicine is about forestalling death and reducing suffering. But is that the case? I'm not persuaded. Furthermore, it treats organ transplantation as just another therapeutic option, and the problem as one in which supply is outstripped by demand, with a resultant loss of the potential good such organs could do. There are significant issues here. Many are common to costly and scarce 'high-tech' treatments; we need to consider carefully what justifies the provision of such treatments and the limits that ought to be placed on it.[77] The added 'complication' is that, unlike nearly all other treatments, organ transplantation necessarily involves the disruption of the bodily integrity of

74 Rachels, Active and Passive Euthanasia, 63–68.

75 For an interesting example of such a thick description using the tools of phenomenology, see Bishop, *The Anticipatory Corpse*, esp. Ch. 6.

76 Radcliffe Richards, *The Ethics of Transplants*, 175–188.

77 I explore these issues in relation to trauma services in Andrew Sloane, Painful Justice: An Ethical Perspective on the Allocation of Trauma Services in Australia, *The Australian and New Zealand Journal of Surgery* 68, no. 11 (1998).

another person, or that of their corpse. I would suggest that a commitment to human dignity suggests that the burden of proof lies with those who would disrupt that integrity rather than those who would resist it. There are particularly complex and troubling issues here relating to the treatment of dying people and their use as 'sources' of organs for donation, and our associated notions of life, death, medical care and our awareness of and response to human finitude at the boundaries of life and death. These, too, are ignored in her treatment of the ethics of transplants, to its detriment.

Conclusion: why bioethics needs a philosophy (and theology) of medicine

And this brings us to the point of this chapter. If we are to do bioethics well, we need to have a clear philosophical understanding of medicine as a social practice (amongst other things). What is medicine and what is it for? Questions such as these can only be answered in light of a broader view of human nature, human community, and the role that medicine plays in their flourishing. But that, in turn, requires careful philosophical and theological reflection. Bioethics needs a philosophy – and even a theology – of medicine. I will return to these issues at the end of the book and seek to show how the Christian perspective on medicine I outline informs our understanding of and ethical response to them. I don't expect my discussion will lead to greater consensus on these issues (perhaps the contrary); nor, quite frankly, do I expect that I will come to radically new insights. I think, for instance, that euthanasia is morally and theologically misguided and has dangerous implications for our understanding and practice of health care. That is hardly an unexpected conclusion from an evangelical Christian; but I think, as we shall see, that our opposition to the practice arises out of more (and other) than an understanding of the sanctity of human life and a commitment to the Hippocratic tradition of medical practice. Perhaps, however, my views on organ transplantation might be a little unexpected (they certainly came as something of a surprise to me). I have long had concerns about the ways in which 'cutting-edge' and experimental treatments come to be expected as the norm, or at least as being generally available as mainline therapies (if late in the piece). It has for some time seemed to me that heart-lung or liver transplants fitted into that category. However, I believe that deeper philosophical and theological reflection on medicine as a practice sharpens those concerns and raises significant others, such that the expectations and rhetoric of the transplant industry need to be more carefully scrutinized, and our expectations and policies criticized and questioned.[78] But that, of course, requires that we first do the hard (and dare I say fulfilling) work of philosophical and theological reflection on medicine and its goals.

[78] I return to these questions in Chapter 9.

4

Perspectives on Philosophy of Medicine

While philosophy of medicine has received considerable attention, most of this has focused on technical issues relating to medical epistemology and its relation to empiricism, evidence-based medicine, basic biological sciences and their relation to clinical judgement, and so on.[1] Relatively little has been done on broader conceptual questions relating to the nature and goals of medicine. I suspect two causes lie at the root of this relative neglect. First, philosophical reflection on medicine and its practice raises a number of important and puzzling matters of detail that need to be examined, and these, while complex, are subject to the kind of fine-grained conceptual analysis beloved of philosophers. Second, what has been called the 'post-modern turn' questions the possibility and desirability of the kind of grand conceptual frameworks required to get to grips with the questions 'What is medicine?' and 'What is it *for*?'. So to echo Pellegrino's happy phrasing, while there is quite a bit of 'philosophy *and* medicine' (questions relating to medicine and its place within the sciences or humanities and so on) and 'philosophy *in* medicine' (questions relating to particular practices or ethical issues within the field of medicine), there is little 'philosophy *of* medicine' (questions relating to the overarching nature and goals of medicine).[2] Similar observations, I believe, apply to theology *and*, *in*, and *of* medicine (but more on that in the next chapter). Having seen how the global context of medicine and reflections on medical ethics raise questions of the philosophy *of* medicine, I want now to turn to those questions. I will use three lenses that I believe will help us gain

1 See, for instance, Fred Gifford (ed.), *Philosophy of Medicine*, Handbook of the Philosophy of Science (Amsterdam: Elsevier, 2011).

2 Edmund D. Pellegrino, What the Philosophy *of* Medicine *Is*, in *The Philosophy of Medicine Reborn: A Pellegrino Reader*, ed. H. Tristram Engelhardt, Jr, and Fabrice Jotterand. (Notre Dame: UNDP, 2008) 23–48.

some clarity on the questions at stake (and which will carry through into the subsequent exploration of theology of medicine): reflections on the nature of health and healing; discussions of 'evidence-based medicine' (EBM), clinical reasoning and medical epistemology (theory of knowledge); and recent work on the phenomenology of medicine.[3] While this chapter, like the next, will be something of a miscellany, it will, I believe, raise important matters that need to be addressed in developing an adequate account of medicine.

Health, healing and philosophy of medicine

It is taken as almost a matter of course that medicine is in the business of healing sick people, and understanding and promoting health. It is assumed or argued to be at the heart of medicine and as its primary goal by a wide range of disparate voices, ranging from conservative defenders of versions of the 'Hippocratic tradition' to biomedical reductionists.[4] The very terms 'health care' and the 'healing professions' presuppose that health is the aim of these particular enterprises. There are, however, a number of problems with that assumption. Framing medicine in these terms raises a number of interesting questions. I will focus on two: what is health?; and is it what medicine is about? If medicine is about health and healing, then we need to know what health *is*, what counts as healing, and how these notions relate to 'disease' and 'illness'. Like love, or time, or personhood, health seems an obvious idea, until we look at it closely. Indeed, as we'll see, the question of what counts as health and what

[3] While it would be interesting to do so, I will not examine critical theory and its contribution to an understanding of medicine, in part because it tends to be mainly of interest to sociology of medicine, and so mostly lies beyond the scope of this project. For an example of the application of Foucauldian critical theory to the sociology of health, see Alan Peterson and Robin Bunton (eds.), *Foucault, Health and Medicine* (London: Routledge, 1997). For a critical appropriation of Foucault in a broader analysis of bioethics, see Gerald P. McKenny, *To Relieve the Human Condition: Bioethics, Technology, and the Body* (Albany: University of New York Press, 1997), Ch. 7; for its application more generally to medicine, see Jeffrey P. Bishop, Foucauldian Diagnostics: Space, Time, and the Metaphysics of Medicine, *Journal of Medicine and Philosophy* 34, no. 4 (2009): esp. 342–347.

[4] Such notions lie at the heart of the varied accounts of Nigel M. de S. Cameron, *The New Medicine: The Revolution in Technology and Ethics* (London: Hodder & Stoughton, 1991), esp. 56–62, 129–145; George L. Engel, The Need for a New Medical Model: A Challenge for Biomedicine, *Family Systems Medicine* 10, no. 3 (1992); Christopher Boorse, Concepts of Health and Disease, in *Philosophy of Medicine*, ed. Fred Gifford (Amsterdam: Elsevier, 2011); Roberto Mordacci and Richard Sobel, Health: A Comprehensive Concept, in *Health, Disease, and Illness: Concepts in Medicine*, ed. Arthur L. Caplan, James J. McCartney, and Dominic A. Sisti (Washington, DC: Georgetown University Press, 2004).

criteria we might use to identify and even measure it is as important as it is controversial. In Chapter 6, I will focus particularly on Neil Messer's insightful analysis of health in philosophy and theology.[5] These, then, will be initial preliminary reflections on questions that I will address in more detail shortly. It will become clear, however, that the problem is not only with the concepts of health, disease, illness and healing,[6] but (perhaps counter-intuitively) with the very question of whether 'healing' is the central concept that enables us to understand the nature and goals of medicine.

Most discussions of this issue start with the definition of health outlined in the Preamble to the World Health Organization (WHO) Constitution of 1948: 'a state of complete physical, mental, and social well-being and not merely the absence of disease or infirmity'. There are at least two good reasons to start there: it plays an important role in international appraisal of health care and health policies; and yet it is deeply problematic. The historical context and rationale of the declaration has been well traced elsewhere.[7] My focus here is on the conceptual issues raised by the definition and the way it (mis)shapes medicine and the discourses of health.

The first thing to notice is that it aims to be a positive statement. Health is not an absence (of disease or infirmity), but a presence, a state of being in the world. That is itself an interesting claim, for health is not something we normally focally experience, unlike illness or infirmity. Illness does tend to intrude on our consciousness in ways that health does not. Health is a background condition, the 'state' that most of us in general expect to find ourselves in most of the time as we go about our business. Illness and infirmity and injury and incapacities intrude upon our awareness when they interfere with our ability to navigate our way in the world. I will come back to this later in this chapter. For the moment, it is enough to consider whether it does, in fact, make sense to think of health as a state; and, if it is, in what way does it

5 Neil G. Messer, *Flourishing: Health, Disease, and Bioethics in Theological Perspective* (Grand Rapids: Eerdmans, 2013); see also his earlier Toward a Theological Understanding of Health and Disease, *Journal of the Society of Christian Ethics* 31, no. 1 (2011).

6 Dominic Murphy, Concepts of Disease and Health, ed. Edward N. Zalta, *The Stanford Encyclopedia of Philosophy* (Summer 2009 edn.) (2009), http://plato.stanford.edu/archives/sum2009/entries/health-disease/ (accessed 19/12/14) presents a good overview of the issues, focusing on disease as the principal category and analysing objectivist and constructivist accounts of disease.

7 See, for example, Messer, *Flourishing*, Ch. 1.

make sense to see it as being more than, or other than, an absence of disease or infirmity.

The second thing is to note that it speaks of 'disease' and 'infirmity'. This also raises interesting questions; for our experience is not generally one of being 'diseased', but of being 'ill'. And, as we shall see, they are different phenomena, indeed, different *classes* of phenomena. Some have raised questions about whether a 'disease' is actually a phenomenon, whether it is a 'thing in the world', and if so, what kind of thing it might be and how that relates to syndromes, clusters of signs and symptoms, organisms and their function, and the sociology of medical knowledge.[8] Certainly, 'disease' bears a relationship to 'illness', but neither are they two ways of describing the one thing, nor do they necessarily coincide in the experiences of clinician and patient. We all recognize the phenomenon of 'asymptomatic pathology', where a person has an underlying disease condition but no experience of that interfering with their capacity to act in the world.[9]

[8] Much of this debate echoes (often unknowingly) debates in medieval philosophical theology between nominalists (for whom universals [such as 'green' or 'good'] were simply names we used to categorize particular properties of things in the world) and realists (for whom universals were things of a particular kind). Nominalist views are often associated with notions of the social construction of medical knowledge. For instance, H. Tristram Engelhardt, Jr, The Disease of Masturbation: Values and the Concept of Disease, in *Meaning and Medicine: A Reader in the Philosophy of Health Care*, ed. H. L. Nelson and J. L. Nelson (New York: Routledge, 1999), argues that the currency of the 'disease' of masturbation in nineteenth-century medicine demonstrates that the notions of disease and what counts as one are socially determined and evaluative notions rather than 'facts of the matter'. While he developed the idea in relation to moral knowledge, I think John Hare's mediating position is helpful (John Hare, *God's Call: Moral Realism, God's Commands, and Human Autonomy* (Grand Rapids: Eerdmans, 2001), esp. 46–48, 118–119). Categories such as 'red' or 'good' (I would add, 'sick' and even 'suffering from ischemic heart disease') are not in themselves things in the world, but features of our experience of it. Nonetheless, they are triggered by and are crucially connected to phenomena in the world (such as patterns of absorption of electromagnetic radiation, or patterns of behaviour and relationships in the case of 'good', or clusters of signs and symptoms and underlying pathophysiological states in the case of 'sick', or 'ischemic heart disease'). The concepts and categories may be social constructs and, for that matter, more or less accurate; nonetheless, when they work, they connect to something that is true about the world. The fact that sometimes what we thought were real conditions were not simply means we were wrong to see those phenomena in terms of 'disease'; it doesn't mean that the very notion of 'disease' is wrong-headed. For similar points in relation to general epistemology and the role of our concepts in connecting us (however partially and provisionally) with the world, see Nicholas Wolterstorff, Are Concept-Users World-Makers?, *Philosophical Perspectives* 1 (1987); Andrew Sloane, *On Being a Christian in the Academy: Nicholas Wolterstorff and the Practice of Christian Scholarship* (Carlisle: Paternoster, 2003), 196–197. However, these questions of the metaphysics of medicine and its connection to epistemology, while interesting, must be left to one side.

[9] For instance, I was diagnosed as having thyrotoxicosis (Grave's disease) during a routine medical check-up a couple of years ago. I had noticed some weight loss but, being a health-conscious middle-aged, middle-class Australian man, I just thought my exercise and diet regimen was bearing particularly lean fruit. The recommended battery of blood tests included basic thyroid as well as liver function tests, and the diagnosis was made.

Indeed, screening programmes for diseases as diverse as colon cancer and heart disease depend on this distinction. Equally, we recognize the phenomenon of 'illness without pathology', where someone experiences themselves as ill, but there is no abnormality detected on physical examination or further investigation. That may be due to imprecision in our diagnostic capacities (chronic fatigue syndrome comes to mind); it may not. All that need concern us at the moment is that 'disease' and 'illness' are not identical phenomena and, indeed, describe different kinds of things in the world, with 'illness' having a clear and on the surface subjective element that 'disease' does not (at least, it's not *clear* and the subjective, or value-driven nature of 'disease' is not on the surface).[10] I will return to these matters shortly.

The feature of the definition that has received most attention, however, is its positive statement that health is a state of *complete* well-being encompassing the physical, mental and social dimensions of human existence. This is highly problematic given its utopian, totalizing and vague character. This has led to a number of counter-proposals, the most prominent of which is Boorse's notion of health as 'normal species functioning' and his attempt to exclude value judgements from the notion of disease.[11] This discussion is important, and has shaped much of the debate about philosophy of medicine (as I will discuss in Chapter 6 below); it seems to me misguided for two reasons. The first is that 'health' is not a concept or a category that can be defined; rather, it is a portmanteau term that gathers together a number of disparate phenomena and gives them an illusion of coherence.[12] But more than that, health is not the category that ought to control our understanding of medicine, and nor for that matter is healing. If the term 'healing' makes any sense, it speaks of restoration of those capacities that enable human flourishing. But much of that is clearly beyond the compass of medicine, for those capacities include knowledge of the world (the purview of education, I would think) and skills to conduct ourselves in it; it includes, from a Christian perspective, being rightly oriented to God and others and the world. And that, I think, is not the job of medicine.

10 Similar observations could be made about 'infirmity'; but there the issue is that it is ambiguous between an 'objective' observable abnormality – say, someone with a paralysed or missing limb – and 'subjective' experiences that may or may not be abnormal – say, the 'infirmities' of age.

11 See, most recently, Boorse, Concepts of Health and Disease.

12 See also Machteld Huber et al., How Should We Define Health?, *British Medical Journal* 343 (2011).

So, to a great extent, the questions 'What is health?' and 'What is healing?', while perhaps interesting, cannot govern our understanding of medicine. First, because the concepts are vague, perhaps basic concepts or composite concepts, and seeking to define them gives an illusion of unity to what are really diverse and even incommensurable phenomena. Perhaps WHO needs some such notion to appraise the relative value of, say, an immunization programme and a primary health-care initiative, or a maternal and early childhood health programme, in terms of health outcomes. And perhaps that's all the worse for WHO, as the nature and goals of these programmes and interventions are so disparate as to defy comparison. Perhaps the best we can do is to establish some kind of (rough and ready) way of appraising the relative value of relevantly similar programmes (this immunization programme versus that one; this maternal health initiative versus that one). Such measures as QALYs (Quality Adjusted Life Years), while they may serve particular managerial and economic agenda, do not, I think, get much purchase on what we mean by health. But more importantly, 'health and healing' are not the concepts we should use in understanding the nature and goal of medicine, because they capture things that do not belong in what we would rightly see as paradigm instances of 'good' medicine, and fail to capture things that do. I will return to these questions later.

Evidence-based medicine, clinical judgement and medical knowing

A number of factors gave rise to the movement that has come to be called 'evidence-based medicine' (EBM): recognition that 'accepted' practices were not always justified by patient outcomes; a concern to contain costs and ensure that medical resources are used most effectively; and a desire to place medical practice on a secure scientific foundation. It is the last that strikes me as most important for our understanding of the nature of medicine as a clinical practice and a practice of inquiry (and will involve a brief foray into the territory of 'medical humanities'). I will come back to these distinctions shortly, but for now let me clarify what I mean by them.

The notion of medicine as a clinical practice is fairly straightforward, almost banal. It is the recognition that somewhere near the centre of what medicine is about is the engagement of a doctor with their patient with particular outcomes in mind. Medicine is about the particular interactions that take place in clinical situations, interactions that, while a matter of course for practising doctors (and, for the most part, their patients) are, on further reflection, really rather odd. Patients will say and show things to their doctors that they would seldom, if ever, say or show to someone else; and doctors will ask patients about things, and will ask patients to allow them to do things, that they would seldom, if ever, ask on other occasions. Some obvious examples come to mind: conversations about sputum and urine and bowels; or activities such as abdominal palpation, chest auscultation, or vaginal or rectal examinations. What gives both patients and doctors the freedom to do those things (and the associated heavy responsibilities on both sides) is that this is a clinical encounter, with a particular clinical aim in mind. Aims such as ascertaining a person's state of health, identifying the nature of a complaint and how best it might be dealt with, and so on. I will explore this a little more in relation to the phenomenology of medicine in the next section. For the moment, however, I think we have clearly enough in mind what I mean by medicine as a clinical practice.

It is also, however, a practice of inquiry. That term probably needs some clarifying. The notion of a 'practice of inquiry' arises out of late twentieth-century epistemology (that is, philosophical reflection on knowledge, rationality, the formation of beliefs, and so on). It is a deliberately *active* and even *bodily* notion. Earlier notions of reason and knowledge tended to be both passive and cerebral. The account of how we come to know things focused on reflection on the world and an analysis either of the processes of reason or of perception by which we come to believe the things we believe. Since the Enlightenment, rationality has generally been seen as the quest for *certainty* and *consensus*. What we wanted was a set of beliefs that we *knew* to be true and which all reasonable people could agree upon. Then we would have a sure basis on which we could act in the world. Now, as we'll see, both elements of this picture of rationality or knowledge are fatally flawed (there is a distinction between rationality and knowledge, but I'll come back to that and other matters later). For now, it's enough to note that humans as knowers were seen largely as passive perceivers of the world; the only activity we undertook in order to understand was mental activity. This, however, fails to square with the nature of human knowing, particularly medical knowing. In order to know things about the world, we actively engage in activities that aim at gaining knowledge: such as observation, questioning others (by way of conversation if they are physically present to us, or by way of literature if they are absent due to distance in time and space), and so forth.

The notion of a practice of inquiry is simply this: in order to know things about the world, we do things in the world. We are active (and bodily active) knowers. If I want to know the history of WHO and its deliberations, I can look it up in histories, or visit their website, or ask someone I believe is a reliable source on such matters, and so on. If we discover that there is some defect in what we believe (there is something I ought to know about and don't; or something I thought was right but now think is wrong, or about which I am now uncertain, etc.), we figure out what we can *do* to fix that defect, or (and perhaps more commonly) find ourselves engaging in some practice that we believe will fix it. It is interesting, by the way, to reflect on how much of our ways of forming beliefs are not focally in our attention. Sometimes we're puzzled as to how best to find out what we need to know, in which case we cast around for the best strategy to find out what we need to know. More often, we just find ourselves doing whatever it is that we know will help: we look out the window at the weather, or listen to a patient's chest, or ask them about their bowel habit, or whatever. Anyway, the point is this: we engage in practices that we believe will help us understand the world in which we live, and generally we do so because there's some aim or purpose of ours that will be served by that knowledge. Hence: practices of inquiry.

Now, some practices of inquiry are relatively simple or, if not simple, do not depend on larger institutional and cultural constructs to any great extent. Finding out if it's raining outside (surprisingly for London in March, it's not), or whether I need a jumper (unsurprisingly for a March morning in London, I do) are pretty straightforward perceptual practices. I look and see; or go outside and feel the air and the job is done. Other practices of inquiry require large cultural and institutional frameworks in order to get going – at least as they are practised now. Medicine is one such. Medical knowing involves a rich and complex culture, and requires tutoring in certain ways of finding things out. We need to *learn* to take a history so as to focus in on what matters on this occasion (being alert, of course, to the fact that rather commonly the presenting problem may not be the real problem). We need to *learn* to touch people's bodies so as to figure out what's going on beneath the skin (abdominal palpation, for instance, is a skill that takes some practice). We need to *learn* to listen to someone's chest and to gain the background knowledge we need in order to decipher the hisses and swishes and (occasionally) clicks and so on that tell us what's going on with their heart valves or their asthma. And there are larger institutional frameworks which inform that, and more. We learn those skills (note the active, bodily nature of medical knowing) in particular educational institutions that are bearers of both unique and typical elements of medical culture. And we depend on large and complex institutional frameworks for much of the knowledge we use. Thinking for a moment of the Western context with which I am most familiar, we depend on diagnostic facilities such as pathology labs and radiology services to help us 'see' what we can't see or feel or hear for ourselves. We need expert knowledge, people who can see what we may not be able to see, or who can see it more clearly. Medicine, then, is both a clinical practice and a practice of inquiry.

And this brings us back to EBM and the controversies surrounding it. EBM is relevant to both aspects of medicine, seeking a more certain foundation for clinical knowledge and therapeutic action than the piecemeal and often anecdotal nature of established medical wisdom. These concerns are certainly legitimate, as 'established medical (or surgical) practice' may be neither well grounded conceptually nor clinically effective, as is evident in such (now blessedly past) practices as 'cupping' or phlebotomy for fever, or routine partial gastrectomy and vagotomy for gastric ulcer. EBM focuses on the second of these concerns, seeking to establish a firm empirical basis in confirmed clinical efficacy and a clear 'decision tree' for all treatment decisions and policies. It also has a relatively clear idea of what counts as (best) evidence: clinical trials of a particular kind, namely randomized controlled clinical trials (RCT) in which a therapy is compared with either another treatment option or none (whether or not this involves the use of placebos). These studies (with the addition of meta-analyses, or comparisons of different trials and their validity) establish a basis of empirical evidence that helps a doctor determine which kind of treatment is best suited for their patient. The aim is the development of an objective body of knowledge that can guide clinical decision-making so as to improve patient outcomes and develop effective treatment plans and health policies.[13] In a now classical statement, it is seen as being 'about integrating individual clinical expertise and the best external evidence'.[14] There is considerable debate about what counts as evidence and how much particular kinds of evidence should count (especially the role of basic sciences and the importance of RCTs); nonetheless, the key appears to be that objective evidence needs to be the basis on which treatment decisions are to be made. EBM, it seems, has claimed the high epistemological (and moral) ground in current medical practice and education.

There are, however, significant conceptual and clinical problems associated with EBM.[15] First, the proliferation of literature in EBM means that clinicians are unable to rely on their own critical judgement but must defer to experts to analyse and digest the data for them, undercutting EBM's stated aim of reducing reliance on authority in clinical practice and opening clinicians to distorted practice due to the vested interests of those who do the RCTs and meta-analysis of them. Further, RCTs tend to exclude the kinds of patients and clinical situations clinicians are seeking to address. This is especially the case because RCTs tend to exclude elderly people and those with multiple pathologies and medications, and tend to be short in duration, whereas many patients are likely to be in a long-term regimen, and so the benefits of a treatment are often exaggerated and the risks and side effects reduced. Further, they deal at population levels, making the rational application of their findings to particular patients problematic.[16] As Bluhm and Borgerson state:

> This is not to say that medical practice won't benefit from thoughtful and critical use of a wide variety of results from medical research . . . The concern raised here is directed not at a general claim that medical practice should pay attention to medical research (which critics of EBM support), but at the

[13] David M. Eddy, Evidence-Based Medicine: A Unified Approach, *Health Affairs* 24, no. 1 (2005); Eddy Lang, The Why and the How of Evidence-Based Medicine, *McGill Journal of Medicine* 8 (2004); David L. Sackett et al., Evidence-Based Medicine: What It Is and What It Isn't, *British Medical Journal* 312 (1996); present overviews of the movement and its central tenets. Eddy notes the distinction between individual patient treatment and policies, but argues that EBM is applicable to both. David M. Eddy, The Origins of Evidence-Based Medicine – A Personal Perspective, *Virtual Mentor* 13, no. 1 (2011), presents a brief personal account of his involvement in the movement.

[14] Sackett et al., Evidence-Based Medicine: What It Is and What It Isn't, 71.

[15] Robyn Bluhm and Kirstin Borgerson, Evidence-Based Medicine, in *Philosophy of Medicine*, ed. Fred Gifford (Amsterdam: Elsevier, 2011), presents an excellent overview of the movement and the key philosophical problems associated with it.

[16] Evidence-Based Medicine, 215–219.

specific rules tying medical practice to medical research in EBM, which fail to capture important distinct elements of medical practice.[17]

It is also hard to square strict application of the principles of EBM with a concern for patients and their autonomy and values, or the values of medical practitioners. EBM seems to foster another kind of (epidemiologically driven) medical paternalism which erases important personal and tacit dimensions of medical knowledge and clinical practice.[18] A fundamental problem with EBM, however, is the way that a particular kind of evidence (RCT) is presented as being at the apex of the hierarchy of evidence. This is in part because it confounds the ranking of *evidence* with the ranking of a particular *kind* of study, whereas there are good and bad RCTs, cohort studies, qualitative studies, and so on.[19] This suggests that, rather than blindly accepting (or rejecting) the tenets of EBM, we need a clinical practice informed by a range of evidence, including clinical experience, basic science and clinical trials (where relevant), but which is not *controlled* by narrowly construed principles of EBM (population-level, statistically driven RCT). Clinical medicine needs a 'methodological pluralism' in which there is no predetermined ranking of evidence (let alone an algorithm of clinical rationality, as earlier and less critical exponents of EBM seem to imply) but a dynamic network of evidence, including personal, tacit, traditional and experiential knowledge.[20]

Similar points are made by Australian surgeon Miles Little.[21] He acknowledges that there is much to value in EBM, especially the way it encourages careful reflection on practice and the evidence of efficacy, thereby eliminating some useless and damaging treatments. He does, however, recognize that the reductionist tendency of EBM and its paternalism and dismissing of the wisdom of the tradition are key problems with the movement. Furthermore, there is a danger that EBM can become an end in itself, whereas medicine is an inherently moral enterprise, arising out of the value that people

17 Evidence-Based Medicine, 219.
18 Evidence-Based Medicine, 219–221.
19 Evidence-Based Medicine, 221–228.
20 Evidence-Based Medicine, 228–231.
21 Miles Little, 'Better than Numbers . . .': A Gentle Critique of Evidence-Based Medicine, in *Restoring Humane Values to Medicine: A Miles Little Reader*, ed. Ian Kerridge, Christopher Jordens, and Emma-Jane Sayers (Sydney: Desert Pea, 2003).

give to human life and our fear of suffering and death. Indeed, if too narrowly focused on evidence, EBM can ignore the suffering of people (and the inherent moral qualities of medicine), and can dismiss non-tangible subjective and qualitative evidence.[22] Medicine needs some of what EBM has to offer, but it also needs to incorporate that which transcends the physical and material, namely values and relationships.[23]

Sandra Tanenbaum takes this further, arguing that clinical reasoning is a hermeneutical or interpretive enterprise in which uncertainty plays a legitimate role.[24] She notes that medical epistemology has two main rival traditions: what she calls realism (typically seen in 'bench science' and pathophysiology), which aims at certain and determinative knowledge of mechanisms; and empiricism (now regnant in outcomes research and EBM), which aims at probabilistic knowledge of what works in practice.[25] She notes that the latter, while useful to some extent, especially at the boundaries of clinical knowledge, is seen as being (and actually is) less useful for clinical diagnosis and decisions about treatment than is clinical experience and an understanding of underlying mechanisms. This is, at least in part, because of the interpretive nature of medical knowledge and the way that being able to construct a meaningful story that accounts for the patient's condition and their progress is crucial to effective medical knowledge.[26] This is similar to Wartofsky's argument that diagnosis, while having logical-linear elements, involves both the play of imagination and intuitive connections that characterize 'getting' a joke.[27] Wartofsky helpfully picks up on elements of tacit knowledge, the importance of well-informed background understanding, imagination and intuition in medical reasoning, in ways that echo Polanyi's notion of tacit knowledge (as well as a recognition of the non-rational elements in scientific knowing found in the work of Popper

22 Better than Numbers, 104–107.
23 Better than Numbers, 114.
24 Sandra J. Tanenbaum, Knowing and Acting in Medical Practice: The Epistemological Politics of Outcomes Research, in *Meaning and Medicine: A Reader in the Philosophy of Health Care*, ed. J. L. Nelson and H. L. Nelson (New York: Routledge, 1999).
25 Knowing and Acting, 61–63.
26 Knowing and Acting, 63–66.
27 Marx Wartofsky, Clinical Judgment, Expert Programs, and Cognitive Style: A Counter-Essay in the Logic of Diagnosis, in *Meaning and Medicine: A Reader in the Philosophy of Health Care*, ed. J. L. Nelson and H. L. Nelson (New York: Routledge, 1999).

and Kuhn).[28] The limited value of EBM in clinical decision-making is also due to the nature of clinical trials and the highly particular condition of individual patients and the correspondingly individual and particular decisions that need to be made versus the general, sometimes idealized, and always population-based nature of EBM.[29] Outcomes research is both designed for and is useful in public policy decision-making, and is not particularly well suited to the kind of work that clinicians do.[30] Tanenbaum concludes:

> Outcomes research should be given its due. It provides a window on the performance of our health-care system. It alerts us to egregious violations of safety and efficacy norms. It offers the puzzled physician a place to start. Outcomes research is not, however, a new foundation for clinical medicine; it is raw material for the artful practitioner. And its ascendancy is a flight from the real inadequacies of health care.[31]

This debate surrounding EBM sheds interesting light both on the nature of medical knowing and the nature of medicine itself. What kind of knowing is medical knowing? Is it statistical and at the population level? Is it 'scientific' and, if so, of what kind and with what degree of certainty? Is it practical wisdom, and, if so, what contribution do population studies and basic sciences make to it? And what is medical knowledge *for*? That is itself, of course, a contested question, but it seems to me that somewhere at the heart of this complex set of practices and institutions and cultures and traditions is the care of needy people. Medical knowledge is meant to discern the nature of that need, how to care for the person in need, and what, if anything, can be done about the problems they face.

Here we see the complex interactions between medicine as a practice of care and a practice of inquiry, and the way that care both informs and motivates

[28] Michael Polanyi, *Personal Knowledge: Towards a Post-Critical Philosophy* (London: Routledge & Kegan Paul, 1958); Karl R. Popper, *Conjectures and Refutations: The Growth of Scientific Knowledge*, 4th edn. (London: Routledge & Kegan Paul, 1972); Thomas Kuhn, *The Structure of Scientific Revolutions*, 2nd edn. (Chicago: University of Chicago Press, 1970). For a specific application of Polanyi's thought to medical epistemology, see Stephen G. Henry, Polanyi's Tacit Knowing and the Relevance of Epistemology to Clinical Medicine, *Journal of Evaluation in Clinical Practice* 16, no. 2 (2010). For the role of tacit knowing in medicine, see David Misselbrook, *Thinking about Patients* (Plymouth: Petroc, 2001), 191–194.

[29] Tanenbaum, Knowing and Acting, 66–69.

[30] Knowing and Acting, 69–70.

[31] Knowing and Acting, 70.

and even interferes with inquiry, and legitimately so. If (as I will argue later) at the heart of medicine is the clinical encounter, then diagnosis as an epistemic practice is warranted in so far as it contributes to the care of the patient. Thus, if the patient recovers, even in the absence of a definitive diagnosis, then the epistemic enterprise has done its job and no further work is either required or desired – unless, of course, there is good reason to think this might be either a recurring condition or that recovery is the result of a masking of symptoms rather than a 'cure' of the disease. This doesn't 'solve' all the problems in medical epistemology by any means, but it might make what seems like a somewhat slip-shod epistemic practice more satisfactory. This lines up, of course, with Wolterstorff's understanding of our epistemic obligations in relation to our obligations in general.[32] Our epistemic obligations (duties we have in forming our beliefs) are a subset of our general obligations (duties we have in relation to what we do and how we conduct our affairs). Normally, we have a responsibility to do the best we can to get our beliefs right on matters of importance to our life projects. We have no general obligation to believe the truth (and nothing but the truth) or to avoid error, for there are too many things that we could know about, many of which have no bearing on the faithful conduct of our lives. The existence of these obligations (and their importance) directly relates to what we rightly see as our responsibilities in the world, and the relative importance of them. That, of course, doesn't mean that a deep understanding of diseases, and so on, is irrelevant to a practicing GP, for such knowledge helps a doctor pick out the most useful course of treatment; but it does mean that her obligation to know precisely the nature of her patient's underlying pathology is less than that of, say, a biological scientist analysing the same condition – or someone investigating the efficacy of certain treatments, and so on. These are different practices with different norms and goals and responsibilities.[33]

[32] See Nicholas Wolterstorff, Can Belief in God Be Rational If It Has No Foundations?, in *Faith and Rationality: Reason and Belief in God*, ed. Alvin Plantinga and Nicholas Wolterstorff (Notre Dame: University of Notre Dame Press, 1983); *Divine Discourse: Philosophical Reflections on the Claim that God Speaks* (Cambridge: Cambridge University Press, 1995), 268–273, and my discussion in Chapter 7.

[33] I think a useful comparison can be made with the differences between, say, a civil engineer and a theoretical physicist and their knowledge, practices and responsibilities.

Furthermore, it sheds light on some of the particular philosophical questions that medicine raises. EBM often seems to run on modernist scepticism regarding clinical rationality: that is to say, beliefs about which treatment is appropriate for a particular patient and a particular condition need to be proven before they are warranted. Such beliefs are, as epistemologists would put it, 'guilty until proven innocent', and cannot rightly be held unless we have good reason to hold them. That, however, is a self-defeating strategy and has been shown to be both conceptually flawed and practically impossible of fulfilment in recent work in epistemology and philosophy of science.[34] A more appropriate stance is to hold that beliefs are 'innocent until proven guilty'. That does not mean that we blindly accept current wisdom in the face of contrary evidence: I am not saying that humoral theories of health and beliefs that diseases are the result of miasma are sound. There is clearly a role for empirical and conceptual testing of medical knowledge. It is to say that excellence in medical knowledge isn't characterized by the scepticism of EBM, but is a matter of wise self-criticism. That self-criticism is necessary because the knowledge doctors claim to have *matters* to patients and their care, and so we have a duty to check that we're right in our beliefs about what ails them and how they are best treated. Nonetheless, current practice and knowledge are fine, unless something causes doubt. And when either the diagnosis or treatment don't seem to fit, it's time to engage in medicine as a practice of inquiry in order to better engage in medicine as a clinical practice. That's when we check with colleagues known for their knowledge and wisdom to see if they have any light to shed on the matter, read suitable journals, and so on. But here, it is also important to remember that the obligations we have to get our beliefs right are only one subset of our overall obligations, and are, in fact, generated by our prior commitment to patient care. It is not medical knowledge that is our primary concern but caring for vulnerable people. And this means that our epistemic obligations are finite and at times need to give way to other considerations. A needy person requires that a clinician act even – perhaps especially – in the face of partial knowledge and uncertain conclusions. Furthermore, medical knowledge, like all other kinds of knowledge, is

a hunch won't do?

[34] See my discussion in Chapter 7.

defeasible. The beliefs we rightly hold are those that make best sense at the time, those that we are entitled to believe. We are entitled to those beliefs if we have done all that can reasonably be expected of us in light of all the obligations we have as actors in a complex world. And sometimes we will not be able to explore all the options; and sometimes we will simply be wrong. But all that can rightly be expected of us is that we take due care in the forming of our beliefs, and direct our knowing and use of that knowledge to the care of the person who comes to us in need. I will return to these questions of epistemology and the practice of medicine in Chapter 7; but for now, it is clear that there are important questions relating to medical knowledge and medical practice that we need to get to grips with in order to understand the nature and goals of medicine.

Phenomenology and philosophy of medicine

The preceding discussion has opened up issues of medical knowing and how that relates to the actual practice of medicine, which leads nicely into Svenaeus' recent work on phenomenology, medicine and health.[35] The phenomenological tradition has played a crucial role in developments in Continental philosophy and its attempts to deal with the problems bequeathed to it by the eighteenth-century German philosopher Immanuel Kant's (in)famous distinction between the *noumena* (the way things 'really are' independent of our knowing of them) and the *phenomena* (the ways in which we know the world, how it impinges on our awareness and the ways that knowledge is conditioned by the structures and categories of human perception, reasoning, and so on).[36] Exploring these developments would take us too far afield; and I am not convinced that we ought to be controlled by these Kantian distinctions anyway.[37] I will put aside, then, the phenomenological tradition's attempt to find a sure foundation for knowledge in the analysis of lived experience of the world and the ontology of

35 Frederik Svenaeus, *The Hermeneutics of Medicine and the Phenomenology of Health: Steps Towards a Philosophy of Medical Practice* (Dordrecht: Kluwer, 2010).

36 Immanuel Kant, *Critique of Pure Reason* (London: G. Bell, 1922).

37 For an incisive discussion of these matters in relation to theology, see Nicholas Wolterstorff, Is It Possible and Desirable for Theologians to Recover from Kant?, *Modern Theology* 14, no. 1 (1998).

the phenomena of human experience that they develop and turn to Svenaeus' discussion of the phenomenology of illness and medicine.[38]

Fundamental to Svenaeus' analysis is the clinical encounter, that relational experience of a physician attending a person in need.[39] Medicine, he believes, is 'first and foremost a practice and not a science'.[40] Clinical practice is the heart of medicine; the science is an adjunct and is important only in as much as it contributes to the engagement between patient and doctor. He outlines a history of medicine, focusing on both clinical practice and the growth in the body of medical science and technology.[41] The development of devices such as the stethoscope, thermometer, microscope and X-ray, and the recognition of the importance and *objectivity* of their findings, led to both true advances in diagnosis and treatment but also a lessening focus on the patient and the doctor–patient relationship.[42] This growth in technical medical knowledge and skill has created both success in diagnoses and treatment and many of the problems facing the practice of medicine and people's dissatisfaction with it.[43] While there has been some interest in researching the doctor–patient relationship, much of it has focused on its *instrumental* benefits rather than inherent value or nature.[44] This, it seems to me, is consistent with contemporary instrumental and utilitarian perspectives in which 'outcomes' are the primary concern in medicine as in other social institutions.[45] In contrast to such reductionist approaches, he develops his own hermeneutical theory of medicine focusing on the clinical encounter. He draws on the important work of

38 In part because I think the quest for foundational certitude is both hopeless and unnecessary; in part, because I believe their starting point and assumptions about the nature of human knowing to be deeply flawed. For those who are interested, and do not share my scepticism about the utility of this aspect of phenomenology, see the useful account in Svenaeus, *The Hermeneutics of Medicine*, 75–90.

39 Indeed, Part One of his analysis is entitled 'The Clinical Encounter', *The Hermeneutics of Medicine*, 11–57.

40 *The Hermeneutics of Medicine*, 11.

41 *The Hermeneutics of Medicine*, 12–29. It is interesting to note that he is sharply critical of Foucault's archaeology of medical knowledge, largely because Foucault pays little, if any, attention to the clinical encounter (for this, see pp.28–29). He also perpetuates a number of unhelpful popular myths of the development of science, especially seeing medieval medicine as simply a 'dark ages' for the discipline, and religion and rationality as in conflict (for which, see pp.13, 17–18).

42 *The Hermeneutics of Medicine*, 29–33.

43 *The Hermeneutics of Medicine*, 33–39.

44 *The Hermeneutics of Medicine*, 39.

45 Another of the weaknesses of EBM is its uncritical acceptance of such an instrumental or utilitarian view of medicine and its value.

Pellegrino and Thomasma,[46] although he does note that their focus on *physical* health results in an unsatisfactory attitude to psychiatry.[47] The clinical encounter, while important in itself, is nonetheless goal-oriented: the goal of medicine is the restoration of health, or the prevention of ill-health. This, then, requires him to develop a clear understanding of health and disease and illness.[48]

Svenaeus begins by outlining and critiquing Christopher Boorse's bio-statistical theory of health, noting that evaluative concepts and whole-person phenomena play a crucial role in the clinical encounter. This means they must be fundamental to a proper notion of health in a manner foreign to Boorse's project.[49] He notes that Nordenfelt's holistic, ordinary-language theory of health allows for such an evaluative dimension, as it sees health as a state of equilibrium that enables people to achieve their vital life goals. While Nordenfelt allows for gradations of minimal to maximal health depending on a person's capacity to attain minimal to maximal goals,[50] Svenaeus criticizes his lack of a properly phenomenological perspective on health. Svenaeus' own phenomenological account of illness and health sees illness as a sustained experience of not being at home in the world, in contrast to health which is a capacity to be at home in the world. Illness and health, however, are not intentional states; they are what we live *through*.[51] 'Health is to be understood as a being at home in the world that keeps the not being at home in the world from becoming apparent. The not being at home, which is a basic and necessary condition of human existence, related to our finitude and dependence on others and otherness, is, in illness, brought to attention and transformed into a pervasive homelessness.'[52]

Having outlined an understanding of health and illness, he proceeds to develop a hermeneutical approach to the clinical encounter, drawing on the work

46 I will discuss their work in some detail in the next chapter.
47 Svenaeus, *The Hermeneutics of Medicine*, 52–55.
48 *The Hermeneutics of Medicine*, 55. For problems with this very enterprise, see my earlier discussion and the detailed appraisal of Messer's theology of health in Chapter 7.
49 *The Hermeneutics of Medicine*, 62–67.
50 *The Hermeneutics of Medicine*, 68–75.
51 *The Hermeneutics of Medicine*, 75–118.
52 *The Hermeneutics of Medicine*, 93. His dependence on Gadamer, whose work he draws on heavily, is apparent in this articulation of health and illness. It is worth noting, as well, that his emphasis is on illness (and health) and not disease, largely because disease is not an existential condition in the way that illness is.

of Habermas and Gadamer.[53] He sees medicine as 'an interpretive, attentive dialogue geared towards healing actions', actions that aim 'to restore lost health – that is, homelike being-in-the-world', which in turn means that such person-oriented interpretation of experience is central to diagnosis.[54] While, as we will see, I'm not convinced that the particular phenomenological approach he takes is satisfactory, he makes a number of important contributions to our understanding of medicine. His focus on the GP as the paradigm of medicine, with specialties functioning as partial exemplars of the fundamental structure of medical practice, is excellent and salutary,[55] both rightly valuing a central feature of modern medical practice and reminding us of the essentially *personal* and *relational* nature of medicine in contrast to an illegitimate focus on medical *technique*. So too, his claim that biomedical sciences primarily function as adjuncts to that which is at the heart of medicine, namely, the interpersonal relationship which constitutes the clinical encounter, rightly re-personalizes medicine.[56] In passing, I should note my agreement with his calling into question the legitimacy of 'enhancement' surgery (such as face lifts or breast augmentation).[57] That is, of course, a normative claim; but he recognizes that medicine is a value-laden enterprise with a clear inherent morality; hence questions of what medicine *is* are inextricably linked to what medicine *ought* to do and be, and, furthermore, the boundaries between 'facts' and 'values' are necessarily fuzzy and permeable.[58]

There is much to glean from Svenaeus' work, in particular his understanding of medicine as a hermeneutical enterprise, one of attention and action,[59] and his concern for the experience of illness.[60] Medicine is both a practice of inquiry, a way of finding out about the world, and a clinical *practice*, a way of changing it. There are, however, a number of flaws in his analysis. First, his understanding of

53 *The Hermeneutics of Medicine*, 119–175.
54 *The Hermeneutics of Medicine*, 179.
55 *The Hermeneutics of Medicine*, 7.
56 *The Hermeneutics of Medicine*, 177.
57 *The Hermeneutics of Medicine*, 56. While he sees that they are questionable in light of them not being about returning the patient to health or preventing future ill-health, whereas I believe that their illegitimacy lies in their not being an appropriate way of caring for vulnerable people, I think his basic insight is sound.
58 *The Hermeneutics of Medicine*, 54, 56, 166–172.
59 *The Hermeneutics of Medicine*, see esp. 146.
60 This helpfully picks up on the important distinction between the doctor's perception of 'disease' and the patient's experience of illness, for which see Kay S. Toombs, Chronic Illness and the Goals of Medicine, *Second Opinion* 21, no. 1 (1995).

the interpretive nature of the clinical encounter focuses on a Gadamerian fusion of the physician and patient's horizons of understanding.[61] This is neither convincing in its own right, nor does it adequately address the essential and necessary and inescapable and *morally significant* asymmetry that exists in the doctor–patient relationship.[62] This relates to a more significant problem with his approach, namely, his dependence on a particular phenomenological theory.[63] His phenomenological perspective attempts to establish a 'solid ground for philosophy' in the phenomena of experiencing the world.[64] Such a foundationalist quest for certitude is epistemologically flawed and practically undesirable. Furthermore, the use of a Kantian structure of phenomena and noumena, in which the foundations of our knowledge are found not in the things themselves but our experience of them as a mediating structure between mind and reality, is unhelpful and unnecessary. It is, to cite Wolterstorff again, both possible and desirable to recover from Kant.[65] Equally, the idea that we can imagine an ideal of a kind of experience which then forms the objective basis for our philosophical analysis,[66] seems to me both speculative and personally and culturally subjective.[67]

Perhaps more importantly, his belief that an awareness of finitude and dependence is an experience of 'homelessness' misses something fundamental about the nature of human existence, especially from a Christian point of view. Something akin to MacIntyre's notion that human beings are *dependent* rational animals seems to make more sense; but that, in turn, allows illness to be something that *unveils* a feature of human existence that we normally hide from ourselves, a feature that is not alien to but constitutive of a proper understanding and experience of human being in the world.[68] Our weakness,

61 Svenaeus, *The Hermeneutics of Medicine*, 174.

62 *The Hermeneutics of Medicine*, 147, where he notes but downplays it. I will discuss the importance of the power differential that inheres in the clinical encounter in Chapters 5 and 9.

63 This is apparent, for instance, in his inadequate attempt to account for such as a state as being in a coma, as it cannot count as illness (not being a disturbed experience of the world, as experience is absent); yet we would normally count such a person as very ill indeed. His attempt to deal with that on pp.102–104 is unconvincing. For a general critique of the phenomenology of medicine, see Tania L. Gergel, Medicine and the Individual: Is Phenomenology the Answer?, *Journal of Evaluation in Clinical Practice* 18, no. 5 (2012).

64 Svenaeus, *The Hermeneutics of Medicine*, 76.

65 Wolterstorff, Is It Possible and Desirable for Theologians to Recover from Kant?, 1–18.

66 Svenaeus, *The Hermeneutics of Medicine*, 78.

67 Here, we need to learn from Foucault's critique of phenomenology and its cultural and even technological conditioning, for which see McKenny, *To Relieve the Human Condition*, esp. 209.

68 Alasdair MacIntyre, *Dependent Rational Animals: Why Human Beings Need the Virtues* (London: Duckworth, 1999).

frailty and finitude is an essential, not an accidental, aspect of human existence and our being confronted by it, even in experiences of weakness and suffering, occasions both the possibility of compassionate inter-relationship, and a greater understanding of ourselves as embodied creatures.

Conclusion

There are a number of things to glean from this eclectic discussion of issues in philosophy of medicine. The first is the nature of health and related phenomena such as illness and disease and how they relate to the practice of medicine. These are complex, 'fuzzy' notions that, far from forming a 'value-neutral' foundation for a philosophy of medicine, come loaded with values and underlying assumptions about the nature of human existence and the ends proper to it and are, in any case, too vague to give us a clear indication of what medicine is and what it should aim to achieve. The second is the nature of medical knowledge and how it relates to medicine as a clinical practice. Medical knowledge, like all human knowledge, is subject to revision and is oriented to and justified by the projects in which it is engaged in the world. The kind of knowledge (and associated practice) advocated by proponents of EBM, while of value in informing public policy and critiquing clinical practice, is by itself neither sound nor desirable for good medical practice. Finally, philosophy of medicine raises questions relating to what kind of practice medicine is, and what lies at the heart of it as a set of institutions and in the experiences of doctors and patients. Phenomenological accounts, while limited, illuminate the importance of illness to patients and highlight the significance of the clinical relationship between doctor and patient, and its centrality to the practice of medicine. Such a perspective requires that we place persons and relationships at the heart of medical practice, providing a helpful conceptual framework that coheres well with theological perspectives on medicine and its practice.

5

Perspectives on Theology of Medicine

Introduction: theology, medicine and a 'culture of death'?

This chapter will be somewhat eclectic, for two apparently conflicting reasons. First, there is a considerable literature relating theology and medicine, making any attempt to be comprehensive self-defeating. Second, little of it seeks to directly answer my primary theological questions: What is medicine? And what is it for? As noted earlier, most of the literature focuses explicitly on the overlapping (but not identical) fields of medical ethics and bioethics and deals with theological questions only in as much as they pertain to those ethical questions by way of grounding a criticism of current developments or alternative proposals. Consequently, I will select authors whose work illustrates important matters that need to be addressed when getting to grips with questions relating to the nature and purpose of medicine. The bulk of the chapter will explore Christian critiques of the current culture of medicine and the way it reflects developments in broader Western culture. This will focus on the work of Pope John Paul II, Nigel Cameron, and Stanley Hauerwas as representatives of a range of Christian perspectives, drawing out key motifs as well as gaps and weaknesses in their work. The chapter will close with a discussion of Pellegrino and Thomasma's explicitly Christian philosophy of medicine, as an example of one of the few attempts to develop a coherent and comprehensive account of the nature and purposes of medicine in light of the Christian tradition.

Christian theological critiques of the culture of medicine

Much of the work in theology of/and medicine has focused more on identifying problems with the current practice of medicine and the cultural values it embodies than on developing a positive vision. This is, I suspect, because Christians have often closely identified with the 'Hippocratic tradition' of medicine, at least as it has been appropriated in the 'Christian' West, and see little need to go further.[1] It seems to me that we need to go beyond such perspectives in two directions: first, we need to question whether the 'Hippocratic tradition' (or rational reconstructions of it in Christian discourse) is adequate for a Christian account of medicine; second, we need to go beyond critique to the construction of a coherent theology of medicine in light of the witness of Scripture, rather than simply grafting Christian values onto an existing tradition. In short, we need a Christian view of the nature and goals of medicine that is controlled by the gospel and the 'worldview' that it generates.[2] Nonetheless, it is worth considering both the critique and the understanding of medicine that informs it in order to see what it might contribute to the project of constructing a Christian theology of medicine.

Pope John Paul II and the 'culture of death'

Pope John Paul II has presented one of the most forceful and influential criticisms of developments in medicine, most notably in *Evangelium Vitae*'s attack on the 'culture of death' that he saw as infecting modern medicine.[3] A detailed analysis of his claims and their implications is beyond my scope; but a number are directly relevant to my concerns.

1 See, for instance, Nigel M. de S. Cameron, *The New Medicine: The Revolution in Technology and Ethics* (London: Hodder & Stoughton, 1991), discussed in more detail below.

2 Despite its currency in particular theological circles, I believe there are crucial problems with the term 'worldview' and its use in the literature. I have used 'scare quotes' to signal my dissatisfaction with the term. I discuss some of these issues in the next chapter. For more detailed analysis, see Andrew Sloane, *On Being a Christian in the Academy: Nicholas Wolterstorff and the Practice of Christian Scholarship* (Carlisle: Paternoster, 2003), 118–121; Nicholas Wolterstorff, On Christian Learning, in *Stained Glass: Worldviews and Social Sciences*, ed. Paul A. Marshall, Sander Griffioen, and Richard J. Mouw (Lanham, MD: University Press of America, 1989).

3 Pope John Paul II, *Evangelium Vitae* (Rome: Vatican, 1995). In the following paragraphs references to *Evangelium Vitae* will be by paragraph number bracketed in the text, following the Vatican's own usage.

Central to his argument is an affirmation of the traditional Roman Catholic doctrine of the sanctity of human life, including earthly life. He recognizes that temporal existence is a penultimate not an ultimate good (no. 2); nonetheless the sanctity of human life is absolute and applies to all equally, from conception to death (no. 2, 57, 60, 64). Almost as prominent is his concern with the 'culture of death' which pervades the modern world and is antithetical to the Church's 'culture of life'. It is worth noting his expansive description of threats to life from the culture of death, which includes poverty, injustice, militarism, social institutions, and so on. While having a clear focus on biomedical ethical issues, he recognizes the implications of what Sider has called a 'completely pro-life' stance (no. 3).[4]

Still, medicine and biotechnology are his chief concerns. He sees the culture of death as even impacting (and distorting) the practice of medicine which 'by its calling is directed towards the defense and care of human life' (no. 4, 89). As is to be expected given his strong championing of traditional Catholic morality, he presents a clear description of this culture of death with particular focus on abortion, but also on people with disbilities and others (no. 12). So too, while contraception and abortion are wrong for different reasons,[5] he links them by way of the selfish human will or distorted autonomy (no. 13; see also no. 16). He raises similar concerns regarding IVF, prenatal diagnosis, and so on (no. 14), seeing the notion of freedom or autonomy entailed in these practices as falsely denying our communal nature in favour of the isolated individual and unfettered expressions of will (no. 19), a perverse notion of freedom that also has dreadful political consequences (no. 20).

The culture of death also finds expression in the practice of euthanasia. 'In a social and cultural context which makes it more difficult to face and accept suffering, the temptation becomes all the greater to resolve the problem of suffering by eliminating it at the root, by hastening death so that it occurs at the moment considered most suitable' (no. 15). Euthanasia, he states, expresses 'a certain Promethean attitude which leads people to think that they can control

4 Ronald J. Sider, *Completely Pro-Life: Building a Consistent Stance* (Downers Grove, IL: Inter-Varsity Press, 1987), although Sider is more critical of the 'just war' tradition than most Roman Catholic writers.

5 He argues that contraception is wrong because of its denial of the nature and goal of sex, whereas abortion is wrong because it is the killing of an innocent human being.

life and death by taking the decisions about them into their own hands' but which, ironically, robs death of its possible meaning (no. 15). Later, he goes on to say: 'When the prevailing tendency is to value life only to the extent that it brings pleasure and well-being, suffering seems like an unbearable setback, something from which one must be freed at all costs' (no. 64). And so death, he states, 'becomes a "rightful liberation" once life is held to be no longer meaningful because it is filled with pain and inexorably doomed to even greater suffering ... Furthermore, when he denies or neglects his fundamental relationship to God, man (*sic*) thinks he is his own rule and measure, with the right to demand that society should guarantee him the ways and means of deciding what to do with his life in full and complete autonomy' (no. 64). This, he believes, is unsurprising, for the loss of the sense of God leads to the loss of the 'sense of man' and so of human dignity (no. 21, 22). Life is no longer sacred, but a mere thing; life and death are not mysteries to be received, but objects to be managed and rejected if we so choose. Utilitarian and hedonistic views take over, and suffering is seen as an unequivocal evil, to be avoided and, if necessary, erased whatever the cost (no. 23). In the Christian doctrine of redemption, however, we see again the value of human life, a value received (and to be given) as a gift (no. 25). Medical advances, when rightly directed and developed, and especially when justly distributed, are signs of the redemption of life (no. 26).

At the heart of John Paul II's argument is his notion of the sanctity of human life, which is given extended biblical justification in Chapter 2, focusing on the proclamation of the 'Gospel of Life' in the person of Jesus Christ (no. 29–51). While fragile and under threat of suffering and death, human life is the creation of God and the object of his love; the weak and vulnerable are especially under God's care (no. 31). 'Truly great must be the value of human life if the Son of God has taken it up and made it the instrument of the salvation of humanity!' (no. 33). Thus, life is (always) a good, because, while fallen and fragile, human beings are made in God's image, are the objects of God's care, are redeemed in the life, death and resurrection of Jesus and are offered the extraordinary prospect of the gift of eternal life. Thus, both the origin and destiny of human life demonstrate its inestimable dignity. Nonetheless, earthly life is a penultimate not an ultimate good, and is given that we might use it in service, even self-sacrificial service. This does not mean, however, that we are free to dispose of that life as we wish; it is a gift entrusted to us to be used according to God's good purpose in which the shedding of innocent blood is always a grievous wrong. 'No one, however, can arbitrarily choose whether to live or die; the absolute master of such a decision is the Creator alone, in whom "we live and move and have our being" (Acts 17:28)' (no. 47).

It is clear, then, that the doctrine of humanity is the key to his understanding both of the cultures of life and death and of medical ethics. This 'sanctity of life' doctrine drives his theology and ethics of medicine. This is both valuable and limited: valuable in as much as it is an explicitly *theological* and *biblical* account; limited in as much as it gives us only a theology of humanity and human society, not a theology of medicine *per se*. Thus, he gives us important theological motifs and locates medicine in the larger story of God's creative and redemptive purposes, but does so only in relation to his underlying focus on human dignity. His perspective also falls prey to the many questions that can be raised about the adequacy of a 'sanctity of life ethic' and its practical implications. It is, however, typical of many critiques of the contemporary practice of medicine, especially in relation to matters such as abortion and euthanasia.[6]

Lamenting a lost tradition

Nigel Cameron combines commitments to a similar sanctity of life ethic and to the Hippocratic tradition in his work on medicine. His is one of a number of voices raised in lamenting the loss of the Christianized Hippocratic tradition in medicine.[7] Fundamental to his vision of medicine and its malformation is the claim that 'traditional medicine' has been shaped by a (Jewish and Muslim and) Christian appropriation of the Hippocratic professional ethos. While he grounds his analysis of the Hippocratic tradition in a particular (and contested) view of its history, it is his conceptual analysis that most concerns me.[8] He

6 See the literature on arguments for and against euthanasia cited in Chapter 3.

7 For at least a qualified endorsement of the (Christianized) Hippocratic tradition, see, for instance, Gilbert Meilaender, *Body, Soul, and Bioethics* (Notre Dame: UNDP, 1995), esp. Ch. 1; John Wyatt, *Matters of Life and Death: Human Dilemmas in the Light of the Christian Faith* (Nottingham: IVP, 2009), esp. Ch. 11.

8 Cameron, *The New Medicine*, 24–45, a chapter he entitles 'The Hippocratic Legacy'. For questions regarding the historical status of the Hippocratic tradition, see, for instance, Fabrice Jotterand, The Hippocratic Oath and Contemporary Medicine: Dialectic between Past Ideals and Present Reality?, *Journal of Medicine and Philosophy* 30 (2005).

makes a number of important claims. First, the Code of Hippocrates is driven by a particular moral ethos, one that was initially largely at odds with the prevailing social and medical culture of the day. Second, understanding medicine as having a professional or 'guild' element is crucial to the Hippocratic tradition. Third, this is reflected in part by the Code's being adopted by prospective practitioners *prior* to induction into the guild, and so was fundamental to the learning and practice of medicine. This is in sharp contrast to more recent practice in which a professional code is adopted *after* formal education but *prior* to entering into the practice of medicine; thus, it is grafted onto the knowledge and skills that form medical practice rather than being integral to it. This means, fourth, that the Hippocratic tradition reflects the notion that medicine is an inherently moral enterprise, and that it is, therefore, more than a set of techniques to be governed by a patient's desires. That last element is clear, he believes, given that the Code prohibits acceding to a patient's will should they request abortion or poison. He sees the 'paternalism' of the Code (in which the doctor adopts a particular moral framework in a pluralistic context and does not automatically use technical skill in line with the patient's request) as fundamental to the nature and practice of medicine and its internal morality; this is, again, clearly in contrast to the (now) prevailing view that sees a doctor's role as providing technical expertise in service of a patient's autonomous will.[9]

This tradition was governed by a moral code internal to the practice of medicine; and this internal morality was driven by a sanctity of life ethic (as witnessed in its minority stance absolutely prohibiting abortion and suicide-euthanasia) and a commitment to healing, rather than the alleviation of suffering.[10] The latter he sees as a significant omission in the Code, again at odds with the prevailing ancient ethos in which, for instance, euthanasia was practised as a way of alleviating suffering.[11] Modern medicine has departed from the Hippocratic ethos in its attempt to combine healing and alleviating suffering, creating a fundamental tension in the practice which erodes its very

[9] For this last point, see esp. Cameron, *The New Medicine*, 28–29.
[10] He argues this at length, claiming that this ethic cannot be 'filleted out' of the tradition without fatal consequences for it (in a chapter tellingly entitled 'The Seamless Dress'), *The New Medicine*, 46–68.
[11] *The New Medicine*, 56–62.

status as a profession.[12] Indeed, he believes that medicine as practised in the Hippocratic tradition is *the* profession, the prime exemplar of what makes a particular social enterprise a *profession.*[13] What makes it so is its covenantal character, in which the practitioner willingly embraces a set of commitments to the deity, to their master and to their patients, and does so in the act of accepting a call to the medical profession. It is this covenantally framed set of commitments that both contrasts Hippocratic medicine and its modern alternatives and gives rise to its inherent moral nature.[14] This internal medical morality which drove the Hippocratic tradition with its fundamental commitment to the sanctity of human life found dual expression in the pursuit of technical skill and moral virtue.[15]

Cameron identifies a number of dangers in the loss of this moral vision. Contractual as opposed to covenantal forms of relationship distort the practice of medicine by subordinating the doctor's technical skill and moral commitment to a patient's wishes, making them a non-moral dispenser of technical expertise. The alternative, as noted earlier, is a recognition of what he sees as a justified paternalism, in which there is a *covenantal* agreement which ensures that the doctor will be governed by a pre-existing moral (and technical) commitment to the patient's well-being, not just their desires.[16] He contrasts the development of post-Hippocratic medicine with a future for a faithful remnant who seek to promulgate the Hippocratic vision as a minority voice in a pluralistic context (both generally and in relation to medical practice). This notion of an 'alternative medical polis' (so to speak) is an important task for Christians in medicine to pursue, one that, as we shall see, has been explored by Hauerwas, Verhey and others.

12 *The New Medicine*, 65–67. For more on this, see his discussion of the subversion of medicine in Nazi Germany and the post-war response, the practice of abortion and infanticide and the defining of some as being outside the moral community and the danger of substituting alleviation of suffering for a commitment to healing in relation to euthanasia (pp. 69–91, 92–128 and 129–145, respectively).

13 *The New Medicine*, 52.

14 *The New Medicine*, 50–52, 62–64. He argues that this internal morality, while derived historically from the Pythagorean tradition, gained sway because people recognized its objective, universal value. He also discusses this in relation to recent work on the sociology of the professions. For criticisms of claims such as these, see, for instance, Gerald P. McKenny, *To Relieve the Human Condition: Bioethics, Technology, and the Body* (Albany: University of New York Press, 1997), 108–146.

15 I think this can be expressed in MacIntyrean terms, that both are virtues inherent to the practice of medicine, one an excellence of skill, the other an excellence in character, both connected to the exercise of practical reason.

16 Cameron, *The New Medicine*, 149–150.

It is worth noting that, while Cameron does outline a theology of medicine, this comes as an Appendix at the end of *The New Medicine*, and so plays no overt structural role in his argument.[17] Nonetheless, his two emphases – theological anthropology and a theology of health and healing – are typical of much work in Christian medical ethics. Theological anthropology focuses on the value or sanctity of human life as grounded in our being created in the image of God and in the incarnation of God the Son in human flesh which, in turn, motivates the concern to heal the sick.[18] Healing is, then, at the centre of theological reflection on medicine and is to be understood as the restoration of physical and psychological health in anticipation (but not consummation) of God's eschatological transformation of all things in which sin and all its consequences (including disease) will be healed.[19] Healing in this understanding is always the work of God, whether that be by 'miraculous' or 'normal' means, and is always in anticipation of the final resurrection of the dead.

> Whenever medicine is being true to itself, its calling is to staunch the wound of the curse, to stay the hand of the destroyer, to secure for life all that can be grasped out of the clutches of death . . . And while we rightly maintain that once the dying process is irreversible there may be limits to what the physician must do, his (*sic*) very calling as a physician is to stand in the breach and to deny death access.[20]

While suggestive, this is not a comprehensive theology of medicine (nor does it claim to be one). Furthermore, Cameron's focus on the ethics of the sanctity of life and on healing does not adequately identify the nature and goal of medicine. Indeed, as I have suggested earlier and will discuss in more detail in the next chapter, I do not think that 'healing' is, in fact, the goal of medicine.

17 *The New Medicine*, 171–184. I'm not convinced that he is able to keep his theological convictions as clearly separate from his discussion of the 'Hippocratic tradition' as he believes. Indeed, it is important to note that this approach is methodologically flawed assuming (as it must) that Christian commitment can and should operate independently of disciplinary practice. For more on this, see the next chapter. It is also worth noting that elsewhere he argues for the need for a theological framework for bioethics, but stops short of articulating a theology of medicine, for which see The Christian Stake in Bioethics: The State of the Question, in *Bioethics and the Future of Medicine: A Christian Appraisal*, ed. John F. Kilner, Nigel M. de S. Cameron, and David L. Schiedermayer (Carlisle: Paternoster, 1995).

18 *The New Medicine*, 172–174. This is, of course, in substantial agreement with the views of John Paul II outlined above.

19 *The New Medicine*, 174–180.

20 *The New Medicine*, 181.

Nonetheless, his work does indicate the possibility, even the necessity, of a theology of medicine, its value for shaping our understanding and practice of medicine, and the importance of critical analysis of the culture of medicine and its relationship to broader issues of culture and an understanding of the nature and ends of human community.[21] These are central concerns in Hauerwas' work on medicine, to which I now turn.

Technology, control and power

For Stanley Hauerwas, medicine has provided fruitful soil for theological reflection, and he notes both the possibilities and temptations of medicine in Western culture. His work on theology of medicine exemplifies the key themes of his work on theology and/as ethics: the failure of modernity (especially in America) to provide people with the stories that will enable them to live faithfully in the world; the idolatrous nature of the alternative narratives that shape our culture; and the call for the Church to live as an alternative community, functioning as witnesses to the 'peaceable Kingdom' of God's rule, by being shaped by the story of the gospel and those practices that both embody and sustain it.[22] Modern medicine, he believes, has come to adopt the idolatrous vision of technical mastery that governs Western culture, seeing itself as the custodian of knowledge and skills that enable us to control our destiny and overcome the limits of finitude, fostering the illusion that we can, somehow, 'get out of life alive'.[23] Modern medicine has no coherent story of humanity and human community; the Church needs to furnish communities of moral agency, grounded in the lived practices of the Church, which can nourish an alternative medical practice.[24] In contrast to the illusions of autonomy that control our culture, Hauerwas reminds us of the centrality of suffering and vulnerability to the human condition and that, whatever else it

[21] See also the comments in the Foreword by C. Everett Koop: After Reading the Appendix, Towards a Theology of Medicine, 'one may wish to see it expanded to become seminal to a new Christian perspective in health' (*The New Medicine*, 16).

[22] Stanley Hauerwas, *The Peaceable Kingdom: A Primer in Christian Ethics* (London: SCM, 1983).

[23] Stanley Hauerwas, The End of American Protestantism, http://www.abc.net.au/religion/articles/2013/07/02/3794561.htm (accessed 15/04/15).

[24] Stanley Hauerwas, *Suffering Presence: Theological Reflections on Medicine, the Mentally Handicapped, and the Church* (Edinburgh: T&T Clark, 1986), esp. 1–17, 23–62.

might be, medicine is a response to that vulnerability, rather than a technique to gain mastery over the human condition.[25]

Despite the fact that Hauerwas provides no systematic, overarching theory of medicine (indeed, in all his work, he consciously avoids what he sees as the temptation to develop a system),[26] it is worth spelling out his views on medicine in more detail. For Hauerwas, a key question in medical ethics (and one that a morally fragmented society may not be able to answer) is: 'What is medicine about?'[27] Answering that question requires a coherent story of human community in which we can locate ourselves and which can shape our notion of human flourishing; this, in turn, gives us a sense of the role medicine might play in those stories and the communities they nurture. It is the absence of those narratives, and the coherent moral vision that they generate, that gives rise to the deformation of modern medicine such that technical mastery replaces practical wisdom used for humane ends. 'Modern medicine's desperate attempt to cure through increasing use of technology may be but a way of avoiding the fact that it lacks any moral rationale for dealing with death's inevitability.'[28]

This is in stark contrast to what medicine could (and should) be. He argues that, in contrast to this thin mastery aimed at maximizing personal autonomy, 'medicine was first and foremost a moral practice constituted by intrinsic moral convictions that are operative even if not explicitly acknowledged'.[29] As a moral tradition embodied in concrete social arrangements, medicine properly formed 'is a practice with internal goods and standards of excellence that give it a moral intelligibility'.[30] Indeed, it is 'a moral art and thus deserving of the designation "profession"', rather than a consumer-driven technological endeavour, and as a profession it 'carries the wisdom of our finitude'.[31]

25 *Naming the Silences: God, Medicine, and the Problem of Suffering* (Grand Rapids: Eerdmans, 1990).

26 Stanley Hauerwas, 2013 New College Lectures, The Work of Theology: Thinking, Writing and Acting Politically (17–19/09/2013; http://www.newcollege.unsw.edu.au/audios/audio-archives; accessed 15/04/15).

27 Hauerwas, *Suffering Presence*, 2.

28 *Suffering Presence*, 2.

29 *Suffering Presence*, 4. Note the similarities to and differences from Cameron's critique of medicine outlined earlier in this chapter.

30 *Suffering Presence*, 8. This explicitly echoes Alasdair MacIntyre, *After Virtue: A Study in Moral Theory*, 2nd edn. (Notre Dame: University of Notre Dame Press, 1984), which he cites on numerous occasions.

31 Hauerwas, *Suffering Presence*, 13; cf. 39–62.

That reality of finitude, an inevitable fate and an inescapable feature of human embodied, creaturely existence, is exposed (perhaps better, revealed) in suffering and disability. In modernity and the explanatory systems it generates, controlled as they are by an idolatrous social vision, suffering is experienced as a threat to our autonomy, rather than being an occasion on which we give and receive care.[32] He sees the particular form of the experience of the suffering of illness in modernity to be one in which such suffering is understood as an organism gone wrong; our hope in the context of such suffering is for the organism to be fixed by the power of medicine.[33] Furthermore, in modernity illness is all pointless; that is, it has no role in the developing stories of our lives except as a problem to be solved so that we can express ourselves more fully as autonomous individuals.[34] This is in contrast to a Christian perspective in which suffering can be understood in light of the Christian story, and so we are able to find that suffering has a meaning, a *telos*, in our stories. But this is something we can only discern for ourselves in light of God's grace, it is never something we can impose on others.[35] The idea that all suffering is a problem that can be overcome by technical mastery so as to enable us to take control of our lives again has become both the goal and the problem of medicine. It explains why it is so hard for modern doctors not to treat (especially treat with 'cure' in mind), and why treatment 'failure' is such a problem for us.[36] This, in turn, exposes the myth that medicine is value neutral, a set of tools to assist the suffering. But it is, of course, value-laden, as is seen in our society's attitude to death – as an evil that ought to be avoided at all costs – and its reflection in medical practice.[37]

Hauerwas' alternative theological approach sees care for suffering, vulnerable people as central to the moral practice of medicine, rather than medicine being a quest for 'cure' or the improving of the health of individuals or communities. He notes:

32 *Naming the Silences*, 39–58. This is evident in the theodicies we develop, in which we attempt to *explain* suffering rather than offer care to those who suffer as a witness to God's defeat of evil and death in Jesus.
33 *Naming the Silences*, 35–38.
34 This is echoed in McKenny's analysis, discussed in Chapter 2 above.
35 Hauerwas, *Naming the Silences*, 65–95; *Suffering Presence*, 23–38.
36 *Naming the Silences*, 59–64.
37 *Naming the Silences*, 97–99. See also the insightful and deeply personal account (from a clearly non-Christian point of view) in Atul Gawande, *Being Mortal: Medicine and What Matters in the End* (New York: Metropolitan Books, 2014).

> Medicine, as many of its critics like to point out, may have little significance for insuring the health of a population. (Effective sanitation is much more important for the health of a population than medicine.) But the care we provide to individuals through the office of medicine is no less morally significant for that. Even when medicine cannot cure, the care physicians provide is all the more important.[38]

Furthermore, 'the ability to sustain care in the face of suffering and death is no easy enterprise, for the constant temptation is to try to eliminate suffering through the agency of medicine rather than let medicine be the way we care for each other in our suffering.'[39]

This commitment is, in turn, informed by a fundamental view of God, human existence, community and its destiny – in short, a theology. And so his is an explicitly theological account of medicine, as he believes that theological commitments 'can illuminate the care we offer one another through the office of medicine'.[40] Further, 'fundamental to understanding the moral art of medicine is the willingness of patient and physician alike to be present to one another in times of suffering'.[41] This commitment demonstrates a clearly moral stance: illness provides a challenge for us to be present to others when they suffer, since we believe that 'illness does not quarantine a person from the human community'.[42] But it also speaks of the kind of community and people we must be and the character of the institutions we must have if we are to be true to that task.[43] 'It does not make *some* difference which community supports the practice of medicine, it makes *all* the difference.'[44] And that, once again, is where the Church is fundamental to Hauerwas' understanding of medicine and the practices that can sustain it as a moral enterprise. For it is the Church that witnesses to the God who is present in care for those who suffer and are vulnerable; it is the Church which is the custodian of the narrative that sustains this moral vision and of the practices that form those who are able to enact it.

38 Hauerwas, *Suffering Presence*, 13.

39 *Suffering Presence*, 17. See also the brilliant reflections in Jeffrey Bishop, The Hard Work of Dying: Refusing the False Logic of Physician-Assisted Death, http://www.abc.net.au/religion/articles/2014/07/15/4046423.htm (accessed 22/12/14).

40 *Suffering Presence*, 6.

41 *Suffering Presence*, 6; cf. 63–83.

42 *Suffering Presence*, 6.

43 *Suffering Presence*, 7, 14.

44 *Suffering Presence*, 15; cf. 23–38; 39–62.

This interest in the Church as providing the narrative and theological framework that makes medicine possible has become a significant theme in Christian work in medicine and bioethics, and needs to be incorporated in a theological account of the nature and goals of medicine.[45]

Hauerwas' characteristic focus on the Church and its practices as an alternative community, while important, is also a key weakness in his account of medicine. As is true of his social ethics in general, Hauerwas struggles to explain how the Church, as the embodiment of the faithful practices that articulate the Christian story and express an alternative pattern of community, is able to effectively engage in the world in which it lives.[46] This is, in part, a result of his relative neglect of a theology of creation and providence in his account of the Christian narrative, and so of the inescapably ambivalent nature of human culture. Culture both reflects God's good ordering of the world and expresses elements of true human community, and so can be affirmed as a gift; but it also evidences the distortions of human sin in the embrace of idolatrous social visions, injustice and abuse of power, self-deception and a desire for mastery, and so must be exposed and resisted.[47] Hauerwas' critique of the distortions evident in modern medicine and the way it reflects a false social vision is crucial for a well-informed theological account of medicine; but a broader understanding of the Christian story is needed if we are to develop a coherent theology of medicine.

45 Similar ideas are found in the work of Allen Verhey, Joseph Kotva, and others, many of whom have been influenced by Hauerwas. See: Allen Verhey, *Reading the Bible in the Strange World of Medicine* (Grand Rapids: Eerdmans, 2003); The Doctor's Oath – and a Christian Swearing It, in *On Moral Medicine: Theological Perspectives in Medical Ethics*, ed. M. Therese Lysaught et al. (Grand Rapids: Eerdmans, 2012); Joseph J. Kotva, Jr, Hospital Chaplaincy as Apapeic Intervention, in *On Moral Medicine: Theological Perspectives in Medical Ethics*, ed. M. Therese Lysaught et al. (Grand Rapids: Eerdmans, 2012); Pastor's Role in Medical Ethics, 272–282; Joel Shuman and Brian Volck, *Reclaiming the Body: Christians and the Faithful Use of Modern Medicine* (Grand Rapids: Brazos, 2006); Samuel Wells, *Learning to Dream Again: Rediscovering the Heart of God* (Grand Rapids: Eerdmans, 2013), 55–60, 80–85.

46 For a general discussion of this feature of Hauerwas' social ethics, see James Davison Hunter, *To Change the World: The Irony, Tragedy, and Possibility of Christianity in the Late Modern World* (Oxford: Oxford University Press, 2010), esp. 150–166.

47 For an excellent discussion of sin and its consequences, see Cornelius Plantinga, *Not the Way It's Supposed to Be: A Breviary of Sin* (Grand Rapids: Eerdmans, 1995).

Edmund Pellegrino's Christian philosophy of medicine

Edmund Pellegrino has made a major contribution to Christian theories of medicine.[48] Drawing on both the Thomistic tradition and phenomenological approaches to medicine, Pellegrino and Thomasma argue for a philosophy of medicine that is derived internally from the defining features of medicine as a social practice, in contradistinction to biomedical and other reductionist models.[49] While Pellegrino's alternative analysis rests on a flawed demarcationist understanding of medicine,[50] there are, nonetheless, certain phenomena which are central to or paradigmatic of medicine. For Pellegrino, medicine is an inherently moral enterprise whose fundamental features arise out of the exposure of human vulnerability in the experience of illness and the response to it in the healing relationship of physician and patient.[51] The power differential inherent in this experience means not only that medicine cannot be reduced to a commodity to be freely traded in the market, but that it bears moral freight.[52]

> Clearly, health and medical care do not fit the conceptual mode of commodities. They center too much on universal human needs which are much more fundamental to human flourishing than any commodity *per se*. They depend on highly intimate inter-personal relationships to be effective. They are not objects fashioned and owned by health professionals, nor are they consumed by patients like other commodities.[53]

[48] This section draws on my earlier discussion in Andrew Sloane, Christianity and the Transformation of Medicine, in *Christianity and the Disciplines: The Transformation of the University*, ed. Oliver D. Crisp et al. (London: T&T Clark, 2012), 88–89.

[49] Edmund D. Pellegrino and David C. Thomasma, *Helping and Healing: Religious Commitment in Health Care* (Washington, DC: Georgetown University Press, 1997), 1–12, 26–38; Edmund D. Pellegrino, What the Philosophy *of* Medicine *Is*, in *The Philosophy of Medicine Reborn: A Pellegrino Reader*, ed. H. Tristram Engelhardt, Jr, and Fabrice Jotterand (Notre Dame: UNDP, 2008), 37–41; Philosophy of Medicine; Internal Morality of Medicine; Medicine Today.

[50] Medicine Today, 135; for problems with demarcationist views of science (in which precise boundaries need to be drawn between different disciplines that each have their own unique subject matter), see Sloane, *On Being a Christian in the Academy*, esp. 11–73, 127–128. For parallels with a Christian philosophy of nursing, see Mary Molewyk Doornbos, Ruth E. Groenhout, and Kendra G. Hotz, *Transforming Care: A Christian Vision of Nursing Practice* (Grand Rapids: Eerdmans, 2005).

[51] Pellegrino and Thomasma, *Helping and Healing*, 54–66; Pellegrino, Humanistic Basis of Professional Ethics.

[52] Commodification; so too, John. F. Morris, Health Care Reform, in *Medicine, Health Care, and Ethics: Catholic Voices*, ed. John F. Morris (Washington, DC: Catholic University of America Press, 2007).

[53] Pellegrino, Commodification, 110.

The physician's power – both of knowledge and skill and the freedom to use them – meets the patient's need with the goal of caring for a vulnerable person and, where possible, returning them to autonomy.[54]

> The essence of humanistic ethics is this: particular features of illness diminish and obstruct a patient's capacity to live a specifically human existence to its fullest. These features create a relationship of inherent inequality between two human beings: one a physician, the other a patient. That inequality must be removed as fully as possible before the humanity of the patient can be restored.[55]

Properly understood this autonomy is not that of the late modern capitalist myth of the unconstrained pursuit of whatever goals an individual may choose; rather, it is the freedom to live within the constraints of the human condition as an agent. Furthermore, such care is incumbent on all human communities.[56] Rooted in the Hippocratic tradition and its developments in medieval and modern medicine, this helping and healing relationship allows for the appropriate care of those who cannot be cured – and the refusal to provide futile 'curative' treatment to them – and for that to be done in a context that values the *relationship* between physician and patient for both its intrinsic and its instrumental value.[57]

While an important contribution to a Christian understanding of medicine, there are a number of theological and philosophical problems with Pellegrino's account of medicine. The first, as noted earlier, is that his analysis rests on a flawed demarcationist understanding of medicine in which he seeks to identify

54 Pellegrino and Thomasma, *Helping and Healing*, 13–38; Pellegrino, Humanistic Basis of Professional Ethics, 93–99; cf. Miles Little and Stephen Leeder, Logic, Hermeneutics and Informed Consent, in *Restoring Humane Values to Medicine: A Miles Little Reader*, ed. Ian Kerridge, Christopher Jordens, and Emma-Jane Sayers (Sydney: Desert Pea, 2003).

55 Pellegrino, Humanistic Basis of Professional Ethics, 93.

56 Commodification, 119.

57 Pellegrino and Thomasma, *Helping and Healing*, 13–66; Pellegrino, Humanistic Basis of Professional Ethics; Commodification; Medicine Today, 140–144; cf. Dónal P. Mathúna, Spirituality and Alternative Medicine, in *Cutting-Edge Bioethics: A Christian Exploration of Technologies and Trends*, ed. John F. Kilner, C. Christopher Hook, and Diann B. Uustal (Grand Rapids: Eerdmans, 2002); Diann B. Uustal, The Ethic and Spirit of Care, in *Cutting-Edge Bioethics: A Christian Exploration of Technologies and Trends*, ed. John F. Kilner, C. Christopher Hook, and Diann B. Uustal (Grand Rapids: Eerdmans, 2002); Kay S. Toombs, Chronic Illness and the Goals of Medicine, *Second Opinion* 21, no. 1 (1995): 11–19; Ruud H. J. ter Meulen, The Lost Voice: How Libertarianism and Consumerism Obliterate the Need for a Relational Ethics in the National Health Care Service, *Christian Bioethics* 14, no. 1 (2008): 86–93.

those features of medicine that distinguish it from other institutions and practices.[58] 'The *essentialist* approach is grounded in the nature of medicine, in what sets it apart from other activities as an enterprise of a special kind, and defines it as something in the real world independent of the construction society might put upon that reality.'[59] This is in contrast to the prevailing reductionist biomedical model, which sees medicine as a body of knowledge and an application of technique to the amelioration of biological disordering.[60] It also differs from emerging social constructivist views, which see it as a practice, the nature and goals of which are determined by the particular communities in which it operates, a perspective that opens medicine to serving abusive and oppressive social ends, such as torture or execution.[61] While it is important to understand the nature of medicine as a social practice, this need not require that it be clearly delineated from other disciplines – a difficult or impossible task, I would suggest. (Where are the sharp boundaries between palliative care medicine and nursing, or between rehabilitation medicine and occupational and physiotherapy?) His concern for disciplinary purity and the precise identification of boundaries is the result of a flawed Enlightenment epistemology; all that is required for medicine to count as a discrete practice is that there be certain phenomena and disciplines which are central to or paradigmatic of medicine. And in that regard his focus on the clinical encounter is valuable.[62]

Clearly, Pellegrino wants philosophy of medicine to emerge from medicine as a practice, especially (the phenomenology of) the clinical relationship.

58 Note the concerns Svenaeus raises about their exclusion of psychiatry from a theology of medicine; Frederik Svenaeus, *The Hermeneutics of Medicine and the Phenomenology of Health: Steps Towards a Philosophy of Medical Practice* (Dordrecht: Kluwer, 2010), 55.

59 Pellegrino, Medicine Today, 135.

60 Medicine Today, 127–130.

61 Medicine Today, 137–139. It is important to note that he rightly contrasts immanent goals with transcendant *teloi*, the latter fitting a properly teleological account of human existence, rather than a narrowly utilitarian one (Medicine Today, 130–131). It is tragically instructive to note the legitimacy of such concerns about social-constructivist approaches to medicine (or radically communitarian ones, for that matter) in light of the complicity of doctors in both capital punishment and the torture of suspected terrorists in recent US history. See, for instance, http://physiciansforhumanrights.org/issues/torture/us-torture/ (accessed 22/12/14); http://physiciansforhumanrights.org/press/press-releases/physicians-for-human-rights-comments-on-oklahoma-execution.html (accessed 22/12/14).

62 See also Svenaeus, *The Hermeneutics of Medicine*, 11–57, esp. pp.52–55 where he explicitly draws on the work of Pellegrino and Thomasma in developing his own account of medicine as clinical practice.

While he sees the need for a Christian vision to inform the practice of medicine, especially in a biotechnological world which leaves us 'abandoned to a plethora of means and a poverty of ends,'[63] this is largely overlaid on an understanding of medicine that he sees as emerging by way of reflection on its phenomenology as a social practice.[64] This is, in part, a consequence of his Thomistic approach to theology and philosophy which sees theology as building on and completing the insights of philosophy *per se*, rather than seeing the belief content of Christian commitment as intrinsic to the task of Christian reflection on medicine (or any other discipline, for that matter).[65] While there is some truth in this claim, it relies on a particular understanding of medicine as a practice, even the primacy of the healing relationship, which is derived from or coheres with, a bigger vision of human life, one that ought to be explicitly articulated in the development of the theory. The dependence of an understanding of medicine on an underlying philosophical and moral vision is not peculiar to *Christian* theorists: all understandings of disciplines such as medicine are informed by and are expressions of a particular belief system.[66] My point, rather, is that a Christian theory of medicine ought to be explicitly and unambiguously Christian, even theological, from the outset, rather than that being an appendix to an account which will, as a result, be driven by unstated commitments that may not be subjected to adequate critical scrutiny.

Finally, there is his view that healing is central to the practice of medicine and health is its goal. Following Galen, Pellegrino and Thomasma define health as 'that state in which we feel able to do the things that we wish to do with a minimum of pain and discomfort.'[67] This is primarily a subjective sense of health vs disease: health is a matter of the integrity of our body and its functions such that we are able to act in line with our purposes; illness is a matter of disunity such that the body becomes a thing which takes over the centre of our awareness and does not function as we wish, thereby reducing our ability to

[63] Pellegrino and Thomasma, *Helping and Healing*, 4.
[64] See, for instance, *Helping and Healing*, 13–38, 54–66; cf. 39–53, 67–83; Pellegrino, Philosophy of Medicine, 51–52; Internal Morality of Medicine, 62–84.
[65] Pellegrino and Thomasma, *Helping and Healing*, 1, 67–83.
[66] Nicholas Wolterstorff, *Reason within the Bounds of Religion*, 2nd edn. (Grand Rapids: Eerdmans, 1984); Sloane, *On Being a Christian in the Academy*, esp. 111–254.
[67] Pellegrino and Thomasma, *Helping and Healing*, 15.

live a full human existence.[68] Illness interferes with human flourishing; health is an essential component of it or requirement for it: 'health, or at least freedom from acute or chronic pain, disability, or disease, is a condition of human flourishing. Human beings cannot attain their fullest potential without some significant measure of health.... It is, to be sure, not the only human good... But other goods, like happiness, wealth, friends, career, etc, are compromised or even impossible without health.'[69] Christianity contributes to our understanding of both suffering and healing: in suffering, people experience finitude and a sense of mortality, vulnerability, dissolution or fracturing of personhood, and disruption of relationships. In each of these, God's healing power is available.[70] Health and healing are, then, holistic in nature, and are not reducible to mere biotechnical phenomena. 'Medicine uses scientific knowledge for its own specific ends, which are healing, helping, curing, and preventing illness and disease and promoting health, i.e., the optimum well-functioning of the whole human organism or human society.'[71] 'The concept of wholeness, together with its asymptotic attainment through relationships between, and among, persons is the specific end of medicine.'[72] There are, I believe, crucial problems with the notion of 'health' and with seeing healing as central to medicine and so health as its goal. I think an important distinction needs to be made between flourishing and health. We have an integrated and holistic notion of human life and flourishing which includes social, personal, economic, physical, mental and spiritual elements; furthermore, health and associated medical care are important for flourishing. This, however, entails holistic notions neither of health nor of medicine. These, of course, are matters that I have raised earlier in this book. It is time now to face them squarely, which brings me to the next chapter in which I discuss Neil Messer's important discussion of theology of health and the difficulties associated with it.

68 *Helping and Healing*, 15–16; 20–23. It is not, however, purely subjective, as there are real ends of human existence that medicine must serve, for which see Pellegrino, Internal Morality of Medicine, 75–76; Humanistic Basis of Professional Ethics, 94–97. See also Svenaeus' work in the previous chapter.

69 Commodification, 119.

70 Pellegrino and Thomasma, *Helping and Healing*, 45–50.

71 Pellegrino, What the Philosophy *of* Medicine *Is*, 37.

72 What the Philosophy *of* Medicine *Is*, 40.

6

Finding the Target: Messer's Theology of Health

Health, healing and their relationship to medicine have been a recurring theme throughout this discussion. Neil Messer has recently published an important book on theology of health. Before outlining my own approach to philosophy and theology of medicine, I need to examine his work, both because it helpfully informs much of the discussion which follows, but also to show where I part company with him.

Philosophy of health

As do many discussions of health, Messer begins with the (in)famous WHO definition in the preamble to its constitution, and Boorse's alternative biomedical theory. Given that Article 1 states that the aim of WHO is 'the attainment by all peoples of the highest possible level of health,' it saw it necessary to define what health is.[1] Thus: 'Health is a state of complete physical, mental and social well-being and not merely the absence of disease or infirmity. The enjoyment of the highest attainable standard of health is one of the fundamental rights of every human being without distinction of race, religion, political belief, economic or social condition . . . [and so] Governments have a responsibility for the health of their peoples which can be fulfilled only by the provision of adequate health and social measures.'[2] While this definition has controlled both WHO and many international health projects, it is deeply

1 World Health Organization, Basic Documents (Geneva, 2009), 2.
2 Basic Documents, 1.

flawed conceptually and open to abuse practically; so too are attempts to expand and improve upon the 'biomedical' model in relation to 'bio-psycho-social (and spiritual)' understandings of medicine.[3] Conceptually, the definition claims too much and does so in such a way as to render it ineffective. Everything seems to count as a dimension of health; in which case, what distinguishes health from other aspects of human flourishing and other demands on social resources? The definition is rendered void for vagueness. But it is also utopian; for what counts as 'total health', and who could possibly claim to have attained it? Furthermore, it runs the risk of turning health into a 'totalizing discourse': that is, all aspects of human well-being come under the purview of health care and subject to both medicine's 'disciplinary power' and governmental policies.[4] The result is that such elements as 'spirituality' come to be seen as measurable outcomes so that when other indicators of health are invalid, such as in disability or terminal illness, these 'aspects of health' can be managed so as to demonstrate the efficacy of particular interventions.[5] As is so often the case, utopian dream can become dystopian nightmare.

In an attempt to avoid the (perceived and real) excesses of WHO definition and in line with the growing 'biomedical' model of health, others sought to both restrict the notion of health and to exclude all evaluative elements from it. Christopher Boorse has in a manner as (in)famous as that of the WHO definition, proposed a 'value-free, biostatistical' model of health.[6] Fundamental to his theory is the distinction between 'disease' (a non-evaluative objective departure from proper species functioning) and 'illness' (an evaluative notion

[3] George L. Engel, The Need for a New Medical Model: A Challenge for Biomedicine, *Family Systems Medicine* 10, no. 3 (1992). It is worth noting that this is developed in relation to psychiatry, which is a particular target of Boorse's biostatistical model and relates, I believe, to a problem endemic to demarcationist approaches to scientific and other disciplines (for which, see my discussion of Pellegrino in Chapter 5).

[4] See Neil G. Messer, *Flourishing: Health, Disease, and Bioethics in Theological Perspective* (Grand Rapids: Eerdmans, 2013), 2–5.

[5] For a stringent critique of this, see Jeffrey P. Bishop, *The Anticipatory Corpse: Medicine, Power and the Care of the Dying* (Notre Dame, IN: UNDP, 2011), 253–284; and for crucial flaws in the underlying epistemology and understanding of 'religion' in much of the literature on 'spirituality' and health, see Daniel E. Hall, Harold G. Koenig, and Keith G. Meador, Conceptualizing 'Religion': How Language Shapes and Constrains Knowledge in the Study of Religion and Health, *Perspectives in Biology and Medicine* 47, no. 3 (2004).

[6] Christopher Boorse, On the Distinction between Disease and Illness, in *Meaning and Medicine: A Reader in the Philosophy of Health Care*, ed. J. L. Nelson and H. L. Nelson (New York: Routledge, 1999). It is worth noting that he develops this account in part in order to ground his criticism of psychiatry.

which relates to 'a relatively serious disease with incapacitating effects that make it undesirable').[7] While there are useful elements in this, evaluative notions are necessary in disease description, in that the goal-directed nature of individual systems cannot be described reductionistically without reference to evaluative notions of the overall *teloi* (ends and goals) of human existence,[8] and non-evaluative, objective understandings of what counts as 'undesirable' need to inform the notion of illness. That is to say, Boorse cannot quarantine the 'objective' and value-free domain of 'disease' from the 'subjective' and value-laden domain of 'illness'.[9] So, while a Christian account of health needs to learn from him, especially his recognition of the limited scope of health as one of a number of goods that contribute to human flourishing, his account is unsatisfactory as it stands.

Messer surveys a number of attempts to navigate between these extremes, ranging from holistic, goal-oriented views of health, through phenomenological accounts of illness to explicitly teleological accounts of health.[10] His analysis is insightful and comprehensive, and so I need not repeat it; but a number of his observations along the way are worth noting. The first is that 'categories such as "disease" and "disorder" seem to have irreducibly fuzzy boundaries',[11] and so while they are real phenomena, we identify instances of them in light of their similarity to paradigm examples rather than their conformity to tight definitions. Second, theories of health suffer from a characteristically modern malaise in which 'facts' and 'values' are seen to operate in separate realms: the first public, shared, objective and rational; the second private, subjective and irrational or non-rational. This is associated with the exclusion of final causes from rational explanations; reason and science deal only with efficient causation.[12] The alternative is to construct an explicitly value-laden account of health in which an overarching understanding of human life and flourishing,

[7] On the Distinction between Disease and Illness, 20–21.

[8] What he sees as the 'apical goals of survival and reproduction' seems to entail that we see them as good things, not just things that organisms tend towards.

[9] See Messer, *Flourishing*, 6–10, for these, and other criticisms of Boorse's theory, especially his (flawed) attempt to separate 'fact' from 'value' in typical modernist fashion.

[10] *Flourishing*, 10–48.

[11] *Flourishing*, 38. I would add 'health' and 'illness' and 'disability' to his list.

[12] *Flourishing*, 47, 50; it is also associated with flawed attempts to clearly distinguish between 'disease' and 'illness'. For more on the reduction of explanation to efficient causation, see Bishop, *The Anticipatory Corpse*, 1–118.

and the *teloi* to which it tends, plays a crucial role. How to formulate that and avoid falling into the totalizing trap of the WHO definition or bio-psycho-social-spiritual accounts of health and medicine is tricky; whether that can be done without invoking a metaphysic of humanity (and the world and God) is another matter. This relates to a third point: a Christian (and so theological) account of health must be related to an understanding of the nature and destiny of humanity and human community and so of human flourishing. Hence an account of health is necessarily teleological in the strictest sense.[13] It is also, finally, a practical concern, as concepts of health are meant to contribute to the practice of health care, and reflection on bioethics.[14] This raises an important question for a Christian understanding of medicine. It may well be that health and disease are important concepts to clarify for bioethical purposes, analyses of social policies, and so on. However, I'm not convinced that seeking to define health and disease and illness and so on is either necessary or helpful for philosophy of medicine (other than, I suppose, demonstrating the weaknesses and dangers of focusing on theories of health in order to understand medicine).[15]

Disability theory also raises important questions relating to frailty, limitation, vulnerability and suffering that are frequently ignored in discussions of healing and medicine.[16] Messer presents a detailed and sensitive treatment of disability theory, focusing on the contrasting social and socio-medical models, and noting the way disability theory raises important questions for any account of health and healing. The social model generally distinguishes between impairment – limitations in functional or cognitive capacity – and disability – a social phenomenon of exclusion and disadvantage – seeing the primary problem as being the social conditions that turn impairment into

13 Messer, *Flourishing*, 49, and this must recognize the transcendent nature of the goods and goals required for human flourishing as the kind of creatures that we are. For the distinction between the merely *consequentialist* and the properly *teleological* (the latter requiring an account of transcendent ends not just immanent goals), see Oliver O'Donovan, *Resurrection and Moral Order: An Outline for Evangelical Ethics*, 2nd edn. (Grand Rapids: Eerdmans, 1994), 187–188.

14 Messer, *Flourishing*, 50.

15 I will discuss this further later in this chapter and in Chapter 8.

16 Messer, *Flourishing*, 50. It is worth noting, in passing, that Hauerwas is a clear exception to this rule – as, for that matter, is Pope John Paul II (for which, see Stanley Hauerwas, *Suffering Presence: Theological Reflections on Medicine, the Mentally Handicapped, and the Church* (Edinburgh: T&T Clark, 1986), and my discussion in Chapter 5).

disability.[17] The socio-medical model sees disability as a result of the interplay of physical and contextual phenomena: most recent versions argue that impairment (a physical, functional incapacity) limits activity (limited activity is what was previously called disability) and restricts participation in community (restricted community participation is what was previously called handicap).[18] A key concern in his discussion is an exploration of the relationship 'which goes beyond a mere negotiation of boundaries, between accounts of health and disease (on the one hand) and impairment and disability (on the other)'.[19] One important area of intersection is between notions of quality of life and disability, especially in the way that QALYs are used in health measurement to the disadvantage of people with disabilities, and the way it presumes a particular view of 'normal' and of the relative (dis)value of disabled life.[20] Implicit or explicit notions of 'health' and disability clearly impact on social policy and the distribution of the resources of particular communities. Equally important is the way that disability and disability theory raise questions about teleology, the nature of human flourishing and the goods of a human life, all matters that have particular importance for a theological account of health.[21]

While all of this is helpful, there is one point on which I think Messer needs to be challenged. It is important to recognize the way that social arrangements, policies, attitudes and so on, can exclude disabled people from fuller experiences of life and community and have done so. Nonetheless, functional incapacity still matters, including in relation to such contested areas as deafness.[22] Here the rhetoric of the Deaf community, which sees itself as a unique (cultural and) linguistic group such that medical and surgical attempts to correct deafness in children are assaults on their (community) identity, seems to miss an important

17 Messer, *Flourishing*, 55–66. He discusses a range of criticisms and developments of social models, many of which seek to ensure that disability theory includes discussion of both impairment (however that is understood and identified) and disability (however that is socially mediated and experienced).

18 *Flourishing*, 67–79. He discusses the development of the model in light of criticisms of earlier versions, especially by disability activists.

19 *Flourishing*, 79.

20 *Flourishing*, 84–86. See also his discussion of cognitive impairment and the valorizing of the autonomous rational self as the key determiner of value and even personhood (89–92).

21 *Flourishing*, 94–101.

22 This is one aspect of disability that Messer does not seem to acknowledge as clearly as he should. See, for instance, *Flourishing*, 82, 84, 98, 100.

point. Deafness is not just an occasion for the development and use of a particular (signed) language, it is also something that interferes with people's ability to navigate the physical world. Sound is not only used for communication and other cultural functions, it is also a way of gathering information about the world, some of which is necessary for survival. The sound of an oncoming bus (or avalanche, I suppose) warns one with inattentive gaze of imminent danger. The world is not just a social construct or cultural product, and we are not only users of language and navigators of culture; the world is a real physical space and we have capacities that enable us to navigate our way in that physical space. Disability names not merely a cultural phenomenon but a real physical impediment, not all of which can be overcome by changing social arrangements. Now, Messer does clearly acknowledge that impairment is real and disability is not simply a social construct; nonetheless, his tacit endorsement of Deaf criticisms of medical intervention runs the risk of the ironic devaluing of the body in favour of personal and cultural choice (a form of voluntarist post/modern Gnosticism), all of which is quite alien to his project.

Despite these caveats, disability raises interesting and important questions for our understanding of health, and contributes to my sense that it is not the most useful category by which to define medicine. For instance: what does it mean to be healthy? It makes sense, for instance, to speak of someone who is disabled but healthy. For example, in many senses, an elite paralympian is clearly healthier than most: the cardiopulmonary function and stamina of, say, a wheelchair rugby player is greater than mine as an academic in his 50s. Yet in another sense most able-bodied people are healthier than a paralympian: a wheelchair athlete, for instance, has little or no ability to walk, and may have limited bowel and bladder control (depending on the nature of their impairment). Such physical realities not only interfere with current functional capacities, they also have immediate and long-term effects on bodily function (pressure care, cardiovascular effects of limited venous return, increased risk of infections of various kinds, all come to mind). Once their condition is irreversible (be that by way of injury or birth defect), it cannot be the goal of medicine to restore that function; and yet, disabled people also fall ill, and when they do, it is medicine's goal to care for them in their illness and, where possible, restore them to 'health'.

This raises, I believe, important issues in relation to health, the extent to which it is a definable or even readily describable phenomenon, and what role it ought to play in our understanding of medicine and its goals. If medicine can be seen as being *related to* but not *about* health (that is, health and healing are not the specific goals of medicine), I think a number of conceptual issues can be resolved or even avoided (cutting a conceptual Gordian knot, or making an end run around a philosophical Maginot Line, perhaps?). Disability and illness are experiences or forms of life in which human vulnerability is experienced and exposed, either reversibly (for some, but not all illnesses) or irreversibly (for some illnesses, and all disability). Medicine is about caring for people in that vulnerability, while recognizing that weakness, dependence and finitude are inherent to the human condition.[23]

Theology of health

Messer aims to develop an account of health from an explicitly Christian perspective, in order to illuminate ethical reflection on health care and so make explicit the assumptions regarding health, illness and disease that inform bioethics.[24] His theological account draws on recent work on philosophy of health, which, as we've seen, is where he begins his discussion. This is not driven by Thomistic forms of rationality which treat philosophy and reason as the foundations on which later theological analysis is built;[25] rather, he sees theology as integral to the task of Christian reflection on health, but believes that it needs to learn from philosophical accounts even as it critically engages with them.[26] However, 'The task of such a theological engagement on the topic

23 And not just, I would add, the fallen human condition, as even in the *eschaton* (the final goal of all things in a new heaven and earth) we will be limited creatures absolutely dependent on the God who has created and saved and transformed us; and this is a matter for trust and delight not lament. While the leaves of that tree are for the healing of the nations (Rev. 22:3), they are not for the transcending of creaturely finitude.

24 Messer, *Flourishing*, xi. He is explicit not only about his being a *Christian* account, but also its being a Christian account of a particular kind, operating out of the Reformed and Anabaptist theological traditions.

25 There are legitimate questions as to whether this is, in fact, what Aquinas was doing, for which see Nicholas Wolterstorff, The Migration of the Theistic Arguments: From Natural Theology to Evidentialist Apologetics, in *Rationality, Religious Belief, and Moral Commitment* (Ithaca: Cornell University Press, 1986); nonetheless, it is how he is normally understood, and is the approach that has largely driven the Thomistic tradition, as evident, say, in Pellegrino's work.

26 Messer, *Flourishing*, xiv, xv, 48–50, 103–107, 163, 210.

of health, disease, and illness is not merely to try to answer the questions as they are framed in (for example) the philosophical literature, but to reframe those questions in light of theology's distinctive sources and methods.'[27] A theological reframing means thinking of humans not just as a *species*, but as '*creatures* of a particular kind', thus reconfiguring our understanding of such matters as the nature of human flourishing and the role of health and even suffering within that understanding, and doing so in light of God's revelation in Christ.[28] Messer reframes his theological account around four sets of resources: Christian practices of healing and care, Barth's theology of health, Aquinas' teleological theological anthropology, and theologies of disability.[29]

The Christian tradition of caring for the sick and engaging in healing ministry arises, Messer notes, directly out of Christian engagement with Scripture. Classical texts, such as the 'Parable of the Good Samaritan' and the gospel accounts of Jesus' own healing ministry, naturally gave rise not just to theological reflection but also to practical care for the poor and sick.[30] While there are critical voices which note the importance of trusting God as the true source and agent of healing, rather than medicine or its human agents, the tradition is broadly affirming of the 'use of means' in that work.[31] However, there is a tendency for Christians writing in the area to equate 'healing' with 'wholeness' or *shalom*, such that it is difficult to separate out those elements

27 *Flourishing*, 104. This bears more than a family resemblance to the perspective that governs my project.

28 *Flourishing*, 105, emphasis in the original. He articulates the 'final authority' of God's self-revelation in terms characteristic of the Barthian tradition within which he operates (thus, God's final self-revelation is Jesus Christ, the Scriptures bear witness to it). I believe there are better ways of framing our understanding of Scripture and its overarching shape; but I will deal with them as they arise in the following discussion. For a more general discussion of this, see Andrew Sloane, *At Home in a Strange Land: Using the Old Testament in Christian Ethics* (Peabody/Grand Rapids: Hendrickson/Baker, 2008), 1–32.

29 Messer, *Flourishing*, 107–134, 134–141, 141–151, and 151–160, respectively. Karl Barth (1886–1968) was a German theologian, one of the most influential of the twentieth century; Thomas Aquinas (1225–1274) was an Italian theologian and philosopher, one of the most influential figures in the Roman Catholic tradition.

30 *Flourishing*, 107–110. He explicitly cites Luke 17:11–19, James 5:13–18, among other texts.

31 *Flourishing*, 121–126. I draw the phrase 'use of means' from William Carey's classical defence of human action in the work of evangelism and mission against those (hyper-Calvinists) who saw such missionary efforts as failing to trust in the sovereign work of God – a debate that bears more than passing resemblance to that over the claims of some (hyper-Pentecostals) who see medicine as a faithless failure to trust God. See William Carey, An Enquiry into the Obligations of Christians, to Use Means for the Conversion of the Heathens (Leicester: Ann Ireland, 1792), http://www.wmcarey.edu/carey/enquiry/anenquiry.pdf., available at http://www.wmcarey.edu/carey/enquiry/anenquiry.pdf (accessed 23/04/2014).

that pertain particularly to health care from other aspects of human flourishing.[32] Indeed, many theological accounts of health care and medicine presuppose that the attainment or restoration of *shalom* is the goal of the enterprise. This generates, I believe, unnecessary tensions between divine and human healing, prayer, pastoral care and medical intervention, and so on, largely as a result of a conceptual confusion. It also, ironically, makes it difficult to understand how humans can flourish in the absence of 'total health'; but the example and call of Jesus to costly service and Paul's accepting of suffering and weakness as the particular form his flourishing takes seem to require just such flourishing in the absence of 'total health'.[33] In light of these confusions, Messer helpfully points out that we need to carefully consider the relationship between health and overall human flourishing. Among other reasons for doing so, this would allow us to pick out those aspects of human flourishing to which health contributes and so weigh up the competing interests of the different aspects of *shalom* that our policies and practices ought to further.[34]

Barth and Aquinas: key theological resources

Messer's own account appeals first to Barth, not just because he is perhaps the most influential Protestant theologian of the twentieth century, but because his notion of health enables us to balance competing elements of human flourishing and to allow suffering and weakness to play a role in it.[35] Barth locates his discussion of health in the context of the ethics of creation, thereby connecting it with the call of God and the capacities God gives human creatures to embrace that call.[36] Health is 'strength for human life', which is God's gift but

[32] Messer, *Flourishing*, 112–121.

[33] *Flourishing*, 118.

[34] *Flourishing*, 117–121. He also discusses theodicy and the problem of evil, largely echoing the work of Hauerwas (see pp.126–134). This, while interesting, is tangential to my interests.

[35] *Flourishing*, 134–136. Messer begins by addressing 2 Cor. 12:7–10, noting that while Barth's account of health bears striking similarities to Paul's discussion of suffering and weakness, Barth never explicitly cites it. I suspect this is because of the location of his treatment of health in his theology (and ethics) of creation. This, for all its strengths, is one of weaknesses of the systematic nature (and particular systematic form) of dogmatic theology.

[36] *Flourishing*, 135–137; Karl Barth, *The Doctrine of Creation: Church Dogmatics* (London: T&T Clark, 1961), 324–397. This gives it the occasionalist, even voluntarist, character typical of Barth's ethics. For this, see Donald G. Bloesch, *Freedom for Obedience: Evangelical Ethics in Contemporary Times* (San Francisco: Harper & Row, 1987).

brings with it the corresponding duty to 'will to be healthy', as that enables us to accept God's call.[37] Barth helpfully notes the importance of broader social, political and economic arrangements for health and well-being. He also, interestingly, 'says surprisingly little about what health … looks like', in part because of the particularity of what form 'strength for human life' will take for particular people at particular times, partly because it was taken as intuitively obvious.[38] In my view, that is an advantage of Barth's treatment, as it allows us to see health as a 'fuzzy' notion that defies definition and precise measurement.[39] Messer notes another clear advantage of his account: it allows us to come to grips with the complexity of suffering and weakness and their relationship to flourishing and health. On the one hand, illness, suffering and death are aspects of a fallen world, clear impositions on human existence, evils against which we need to struggle. But on the other, they are both reminders of the realities of human vulnerability and finitude, and the dependence on God that define human created (not just fallen) existence, and can also contribute to that eschatological flourishing to which the gospel calls us and which can be modelled by us as those who live 'between the times'.[40] The way that this is articulated, however, leaves something to be desired.

For Messer, as for Barth, the nature of true human creaturely existence is found in the person of Jesus Christ. While this is a welcome emphasis, it limits the way that the biblical narrative and key theological motifs are allowed to shape our understanding of human flourishing and creates difficulties in the way he accounts for the creaturely goods of health. While I believe he is right to see personal survival and reproduction as relative, not absolute, goods of human existence,[41] his Christocentric focus fails to give due weight to them as creational goods. It is not because human survival is guaranteed by 'new creation' that personal survival or reproduction can be 'trumped' by the gift of martyrdom or celibacy, but because the love of God trumps all other loves, and God's kingdom is a priority that trumps all others (Matt. 6:33, 19:12, 22:37-40;

37 Messer, *Flourishing*, 136, 138; Barth, *CD* III.4, 356–360.
38 Messer, *Flourishing*, 138.
39 See my reflections at the end of this chapter and in Chapter 9.
40 Messer, *Flourishing*, 139–141; Barth, *CD* III.4, 366–368.
41 Messer, *Flourishing*, 137.

1 Cor. 7:32-35).[42] Furthermore, the narrative that climaxes in the person and ministry of Jesus Christ and is consummated in the *eschaton*,[43] does not replace creation and its goods, it vindicates and redeems and transforms them so that God's original purposes for human and nonhuman creation are fulfilled.[44]

Recognizing the importance of the notion of human flourishing and its role as the *telos* to which human life is oriented, Messer turns to Aquinas to supplement Barth's account of health. He recognizes that Barth and Aquinas are generally seen as theological opponents rather than allies, but believes that the teleology implicit in Barth can cohere well with that explicitly articulated by Aquinas.[45] Key elements in Aquinas' understanding are that beings and their histories are to be understood in relation to *final* not just *efficient* causation, and that *form* is important to the ends that are proper to a particular organism. 'In other words, to be a creature of a particular kind just is to be a creature whose good, or flourishing, consists in some things rather than others.'[46] To be a creature of the human kind means to be a rational animal whose final good consists in the beatific vision, the contemplation of God. For the Thomistic tradition this creates difficulties in relation to the goods of earthly existence, as well as overly valuing reason as opposed to other features of human existence.[47] While I appreciate his attempt to bring these two great theologians together, it seems to me that an easier and theologically richer route can be found via the redemptive-historical framework of Neo-Calvinism (and an associated narratively driven biblical theology) and the vision of the Kingdom of God (or *shalom*) which it articulates.[48] But before I turn to more

[42] It seems to me that the reference to marriage in heaven in Matt. 22:30 relates not to a negation of marriage and reproduction in the *eschaton* (about that, I am agnostic), but to the nature of inheritance. The Sadducees appeal to the levirate marriage legislation, in which a man was required to marry his dead brother's widow should he die without issue, in order that his name be sustained and his inheritance ensured. Isaiah 56 already tells us that God's eschatological promises include a future for the eunuch, an inheritance among the people of God. That, I believe, is what Jesus refers to here.

[43] That is, it reaches its fulfilment and goal in a transformed new creation.

[44] See Romans 8. O'Donovan, *Resurrection and Moral Order*, esp. 11–75; Tom Wright, *Surprised by Hope* (London: SPCK, 2007). A more biblically driven narrative approach to theology would allow these emphases to play their rightful role, as I will discuss in the next chapter.

[45] Messer, *Flourishing*, 141–142.

[46] *Flourishing*, 148.

[47] *Flourishing*, 147–150. See also the critique in Nicholas Wolterstorff, *Until Justice and Peace Embrace* (Grand Rapids: Eerdmans, 1983), 3–22, 124–140.

[48] For this see, for instance, Craig G. Bartholomew and Michael W. Goheen, *The Drama of Scripture: Finding Our Place in the Biblical Story* (Grand Rapids: Baker Academic, 2004); Wolterstorff, *Until Justice and Peace Embrace*, esp. 69–72.

detailed analysis of Messer's own views, it is important to note the contribution of theologies of disability to his overall discussion.

Theologies of disability: a key contribution

Many notions of health presuppose a view of 'normality' such that any departure from the normal counts as a failure to flourish, understood as either illness or disability. Disability theologies challenge that, suggesting that we need to broaden our understanding of human flourishing so that divergence from a (statistical) norm is not to be equated with illness or a failure to flourish.[49] They also challenge the centrality of rational autonomy in many contemporary philosophies of disability in light of reflection on intellectual disability and the way that profoundly disabled people contribute to the well-being of their communities.[50] Limitation and vulnerability, normally seen to be impediments to human freedom and so flourishing, need to be understood, instead, as fundamental features of what it means to be creatures of the human kind, and so as not only consistent with human flourishing but, properly embraced, constitutive of it.[51] Some impairments, of course, need to be seen as threats to human flourishing; but inclusion of people with disabilities, including profound intellectual disabilities, also enriches our communities and so, in an apparently paradoxical, but also deeply *Christian* way, contribute to human flourishing. Properly lived finitude is a key virtue, a pattern of thought and affect and life that contributes to the flourishing of humans and human communities. Chronic illness and disability and other ways that brokenness impinges on our lives force us both to confront the realities of vulnerability and finitude in ourselves and others and to allow God's Spirit to form us and our thoughts, desires and the patterns of our lives in light of our creaturely limitations and in anticipation of the eschatological transformation of all things.

This last point needs to be made very carefully, lest we lapse into patronizing sentimentality or naïve idealism. Disability, like illness, is a mark of fallen

49 Messer, *Flourishing*, 158.

50 *Flourishing*, 151–152, 155, 157–159. For an interesting (if overly sentimental) personal account of this, see Henri J. M. Nouwen, *Adam: God's Beloved* (Maryknoll, NY: Orbis, 1997).

51 See also Alasdair MacIntyre, *Dependent Rational Animals: Why Human Beings Need the Virtues* (London: Duckworth, 1999).

existence as well as a reminder of the limitations of human finitude and an opportunity to express evangelical community (that is, community life shaped by the good news of Jesus). It may, in God's mercy, become a 'good-for' us, but it is not thereby a good in itself, a point where I think I part company with Messer (or at least where he needs to clarify his views). He seems to imply that we need to endorse the idea that the crucifixion of Jesus means we worship a 'disabled God', and so human disability will be incorporated into our eschatological future.[52] I am not convinced. Here, reflection on Jesus' wounds is instructive. The visible wounds of the resurrected Jesus are not presented in either the gospels or the Apocalypse as signs of his current disability, the elevation of disability into his glorified form, but of the overcoming of death and of the clear identity of the risen Jesus with the one who was crucified. Of course, the form of the victory of the Crucified One is precisely through (and so over) death; but it is also the victory of the Risen One who has conquered death and Hades and who is, then, the Lord of life. The wounds are fundamental to his 'storied identity', and so woundedness can be fundamental to ours, but this is not an 'eternal' valuation of disability, but the form of discipleship we need to embrace even as it is the form of power that a broken world needs. The wound struck so deeply into the world by human sin is healed by its being struck as deeply in the flesh of God the Son as it was in the world, and by its being healed, but not erased, in his overcoming of death.

A constructive theology of health

Messer's own constructive account of health and disease is outlined in a series of sixteen theses organized under four main headings. The first four theses fall under the heading 'Humans as Creatures'. He begins by arguing that the nature of human creaturely existence, especially as understood in light of Jesus, determines a properly *theological* account of health and disease. In such an

52 Messer, *Flourishing*, 153, 158. I should note, however, his resistance to one-sided views of divine weakness, noting that the Cross is both suffering and the exercise of saving power (see the extended discussion in fn.191, pp.158–159). Nonetheless, I think he needs to be clearer about just how he thinks of the role of disability in the *eschaton*. The notion of the 'disabled God' of the resurrection comes from Eiesland's disability theology. See, for instance, Nancy L. Eiesland, Encountering the Disabled God, in *On Moral Medicine: Theological Perspectives in Medical Ethics*, ed. M. Therese Lysaught et al. (Grand Rapids: Eerdmans, 2012).

account, we have 'proximate' (or penultimate) as well as ultimate ends and goods associated with them; the fulfilment of these ends constitutes human flourishing. The nature of both humanity and the ends proper to us need to be framed in scientific and also in theological terms; but the latter are to 'control' our understanding of human flourishing and so will necessarily include descriptive and evaluative content.[53] Our ultimate end, life in union with God, gives us the fullest context in which to understand human existence, giving an 'eschatological horizon' to our account of human flourishing, and so of health. He notes that the Christian tradition has often over-valued rationality and under-valued human bodily existence (and I would add, communal life and our connection with other creatures), which needs to be corrected in a more satisfactory account of health.[54] The penultimate ends of human creaturely existence are real and universal; while all forms of knowledge can contribute to our understanding of those ends, they are understood in the first instance by way of God's revelation in Christ.[55] There are, nonetheless, particular ends and associated goods that relate to the different callings given to different people; discerning those ends and the means to attain them requires both practical wisdom and openness to the particularity of God's command.[56]

The next five theses are organized under the heading 'Health and Creaturely Flourishing'. While a concern for wholeness and human well-being are important, they are not to be equated with health as is the case in the WHO

[53] Messer, *Flourishing*, 164–168, thesis (i). Notice, again, the importance of recognizing the interplay between 'facts' and 'values', descriptive and normative accounts of (human) reality.

[54] *Flourishing*, 164–170, thesis (ii). He finds Bonhoeffer's notion of the ultimate (eschatological) and penultimate (embodied life here and now) valuable as a way of affirming 'temporal' goods, but only in as much as they find their meaning in and are relativized by ultimate, eschatological goods. This seems to me to fail to do justice to the integrity of creation and its goodness in and for God's purposes. See also McKenny's discussion of Gustafson's theocentric bioethics and the importance of broader creational concerns in Gerald P. McKenny, *To Relieve the Human Condition: Bioethics, Technology, and the Body* (Albany: University of New York Press, 1997), 76–107.

[55] Messer, *Flourishing*, 170–172, thesis (iii). It is worth noting his acknowledgement of the 'noetic effects of sin', as well as the value of human learning, but the priority of God's revelation in shaping properly Christian knowledge. Once again, however, he frames this in Barthian terms with respect to God's self-revelation in Christ, rather than more biblical-theological and narrative terms. These matters will be taken up in some detail in chapter 7.

[56] *Flourishing*, 172–174, thesis (iv). Once again, I note my caveats regarding the specifically Barthian form this takes; nonetheless, the notion of vocation or calling and the way this relates to both the generalities of our common creaturely life and the particular shape of an individual's life is helpful. For this, see also John Hare, *God's Call: Moral Realism, God's Commands, and Human Autonomy* (Grand Rapids: Eerdmans, 2001); *Why Bother Being Good? The Place of God in the Moral Life* (Downers Grove: IVP, 2002).

definition and many Christian theologies of health. The dangers of such 'totalizing' views of health have already been noted; they also tend to limit notions of flourishing or *shalom* to that which can be encompassed in some notion of health, and fail to recognize that wholeness is an eschatological gift from God, not an immanent result of human striving.[57] He argues that Barth's *definition* of health as 'strength for human life' provides valuable resources for a theological account of health. Integration of human bodily and intellectual systems so as to enable humans to be about their business in the world is an important aspect of this 'strength'; but this needs to be understood in such a way as to include rather than exclude people with disabilities from our notion of flourishing and the practices that go along with them.[58] Theological treatments of human flourishing can learn from and incorporate insights from evolutionary biology and other scientific understandings of our physical and psychological functioning, so long as they are critically appropriated in light of Christ. Of particular importance here is the inclusion of questions of value and final causation that are normally methodologically excluded from scientific accounts, but which are necessary for a properly teleological understanding of human life and flourishing.[59] Health needs to be understood in eschatological perspective. He states: 'Health is a *penultimate* good, concerned with the fulfilment of proximate human goals or ends, although it points towards the ultimate fulfilment of human life. If it is treated as an ultimate end – which is a form of idolatry – the results are likely to prove destructive.'[60] He believes that where there is eschatological completion of 'health goals', this ultimate fulfilment will involve 'the transformation, not merely the continuation, of the goods of this-worldly health.'[61] He rightly notes that this is a divine gift not a

[57] Messer, *Flourishing*, 174–175, thesis (v).

[58] *Flourishing*, 175–179, thesis (vi). He does acknowledge that some impairments severely and irreversibly restrict a person's capacity to flourish in this life, requiring that we remember the eschatological context of a theology of flourishing.

[59] *Flourishing*, 179–181, thesis (vii). Again, he formulates this in Christocentric terms; I think a more expansive theological framework is more helpful, for which see below.

[60] *Flourishing*, 181, thesis (viii), emphasis in the original. While helpful, I think this could be better framed along other lines: health or wholeness are eschatological gifts; as such, they are only ever partially attained as a result of human striving, and ought to be understood as a response to God's grace; this means there are crucial limits to what we can attain here and now; only the *eschaton* will see the full realization of God's creative purposes and so the vindication and transformation of creational goods such as health and wholeness. I will take this discussion further in subsequent chapters.

[61] *Flourishing*, 181.

human attainment; when treated as an ultimate goal, health or the extension of human life become idolatrous and destructive.[62] Furthermore, health is a social and political matter as well as an individual one; thus medical care is not the only (or even in many instances the primary) determinant of either health or disability.[63]

'Disease, Suffering, Evil, and Sin' is the third category of theses in Messer's account. A disease is any 'internal state, condition, or process, which tends to disrupt a physical or mental function such that the fulfilment of a proximate end of embodied creaturely human life is hindered or threatened'.[64] This involves recognition of harmful dysfunctions, as well as paradigmatic cases of what counts as disease, recognizing that given the necessary imprecision of the categories, practical wisdom will be required in the discernment of diseases.[65] The complex connections that exist between disease and sin and evil require that we recognize disease as an evil, a sign of the fallenness of the world occasioned by human sin, but also as a mark of God's judgement on it. It also requires that we realize that it is not God's 'positive will' for God's creatures, and that God has acted to reverse it in the healings of Jesus (as well as God's providential governing of the world), and will eradicate it in the *eschaton*.[66] The similarly complex relationship between impairment, disability and disease means that we cannot draw sharp boundaries between them; we can neither treat all significant variations from statistical norms as pathologies nor ignore the ways that social structures and personal attitudes threaten the flourishing of people with disabilities.[67] Despite the fact that disease and illness are not

62 *Flourishing*, 181–182.

63 *Flourishing*, 182–184, thesis (ix).

64 *Flourishing*, 184.

65 *Flourishing*, 184–186, thesis (x). Given my reservations about defining 'health', I have corresponding reservations about defining disease, and in seeing the treating of disease as what medicine is about. It seems to me that identifying paradigmatic cases of human need that medicine can rightly care for may be a more fruitful way forward.

66 *Flourishing*, 186–189, thesis (xi). The notion of God's 'positive will' draws an important distinction between what God positively wills and what God permits. We must also recognize, however, that Scripture records God acting in judgement, including by way of disease (Exodus 7–12; Deut. 28:22), and that God's capacity to both 'wound' and 'heal' is a mark of God's sovereign power in achieving God's ends in the world, in contrast to the impotence of the idols (see, for instance, Deut. 32:39, Isa. 45:7). Neither text, however, should be taken to indicate that disease is always evidence that God is acting in judgement against an individual or community – as both the book of Job and John 9 demonstrate.

67 *Flourishing*, 189–190, thesis (xii).

conceptually distinct, it is important to recognize that patients' perspectives and experiences of illness and suffering differ from that of their carers, which needs to be factored into our account of health and human flourishing – even to the extent of seeing suffering as being transformed by God's grace into an occasion for 'eschatological' flourishing.[68] The 'penultimate' nature of health and human life means, furthermore, that even the evil of death is a relative, not an absolute evil. As such, it must not be treated as the ultimate disease subject to a final technical or medical solution, but as the final enemy, already vanquished in the resurrection of Jesus; victory over death will only be ours as God's eschatological gift.[69]

Given the importance of the *practice* of health care in a Christian view of the world, it is fitting that the final heading should be 'Practical Implications' under which his last two theses are organized. The work of medicine and of healing is clearly affirmed; but it needs to be a qualified affirmation given the tendency to absolutize health and to trust technique rather than God, and the limited role of medicine in fostering human health.[70] Finally, given that cure is not always possible, and death is inevitable, Christians need to embrace the call to care when cure is not possible, and to foster the community practices that can sustain such care.[71]

Messer's theology of health is rich and helpful and provides a number of necessary correctives to contemporary bioethics, not least of which is his explicitly theological focus. It is also important for me to acknowledge that my project is different to Messer's, and so I will not criticize him for asking a different set of questions to mine. However, as I've noted, there are a number of areas where I think he needs either greater clarity or a more fruitful theological framework. I would also like to reflect a little on a more fundamental issue: can the notion of health do the kind of work that Messer wants it to do? Indeed, is 'health' a useful category and should it determine our understanding of the nature and goals of medicine? It seems to me that 'health' is a shorthand expression for a range of disparate phenomena and concerns. If it is used in

[68] *Flourishing*, 191–193, thesis (xiii). See also my comments earlier.
[69] *Flourishing*, 194–197, thesis (xiv).
[70] *Flourishing*, 197–199, thesis (xv).
[71] *Flourishing*, 199–200, thesis (xvi). See the discussion of Hauerwas above.

such a loose way, then it may be useful, but only if that is done without attempting to unite them in one comprehensive concept. Trying to be overly precise as to what counts as health and how that differs from and relates to illness and disease and disability risks conceptual confusion and distorted practice.[72]

To be fair, Messer is clear about the vagueness of key concepts and the importance of recognizing that when measuring efficacy of treatment regimen or health policies it is preferable to adopt condition-specific measures rather than global, generic health metrics. I think that's exactly right. However, talking in terms of health can create the illusion that when examining, say, prosthetic services for amputees, chemotherapy for people with cancer, and dialysis services for people with renal failure, we are looking at different forms of the one phenomenon. While bureaucrats, health economists and others who seek managerial control of the health-care system may value such comparisons, it seems to me that they are attempting to compare incommensurables. When this is allied with particular social and political agendas, and implicit values being placed on particular conditions or ages or disabilities, the risk of devaluing some people in theory and excluding their concerns in practice is almost unavoidable.

I think we need to 'come clean'. Speaking of health in general conversation, and even philosophical and theological analysis has its place; but health has neither the coherence nor the clarity it needs for it to bear the weight given to it in philosophical and political discussions of medicine, health care and biotechnology. Health care and biotechnology are complex institutions and social practices that aim to address a range of human needs that differ so widely that attempts to analyse them using one comprehensive term are doomed to failure.[73] Perhaps more importantly, attempts to determine the

[72] For helpful discussions of these and related matters (if from different conceptual perspectives than mine), see R. M. Hare, Health, *Journal of Medical Ethics* 12, no. 4 (1986); Germund Hesslow, Do We Need a Concept of Disease?, *Theoretical Medicine* 14 (1993); Dean Rickles, Public Health, in *Philosophy of Medicine*, ed. Fred Gifford (Amsterdam: Elsevier, 2011). Rickles adopts a pragmatic approach to health in which he argues 'that it is nonsense to try to pin down a unique definition of health and disease independently of one's interests and the uses to which the concepts are being put. This filters through into the (operational) construction of population measures of health and disease . . . there are many such measures, and one can pick and choose according to the task' (541) and so different measures may be used in relation, say, to resource allocation to those used in relation to questions of equity.

[73] See Public Health, 544–556.

'health utility' of diverse treatments or policies will distort the data and generate unhelpful, even dangerous policies. These policy decisions require clearer articulation of the values that are enshrined in our institutions and practices and the way they reflect an underlying notion of human community (and, yes, of human flourishing). Their implementation cannot be by way of the operation of a uniform utilitarian algorithm but by the exercise of fine-grained judgements of practical reason that, while sensitive to questions of cost and benefit, are not bound by the strictures of health-care economics. All this is obscured, I think, by attempts to develop a coherent theology of health. These criticisms raise concerns about whether we can come to grips with the nature and goals of medicine if we can't come to grips with the notion of health and healing. This begs the question as to whether medicine is, in fact, about health, a matter to which I will return.[74]

[74] See the discussion in Chapter 8.

7

A Philosophical-Theological Framework for Medicine

A philosophical framework: practising *Christian* scholarship

My discussion so far has presupposed that Christian faith provides resources we can use to understand and critique medicine, and that these resources should be used. It is time now to justify that presupposition and make some explicit claims about it.

The very notion that as Christians we can and ought to allow our Christian commitment to inform our understanding of particular disciplines and their ways of construing the world has come under fire from a number of directions (where it hasn't been simply dismissed with derisory contempt). Now, this book presupposes the very idea of Christian scholarship and its need to impact on the disciplines. Nonetheless, it is worth my while briefly pointing out reasons why this project is not wrong-headed, in part because that will help distinguish my understanding of epistemology (the philosophy of belief, belief-formation, knowledge and related matters) from other contenders.

Medicine and epistemology

Something akin to the Enlightenment project seems to underlie most discussions of medicine and medical knowing – most obviously in attempts like Boorse's to come up with a value-neutral account of health and the kind of knowledge valued in EBM, but even in Svenaeus' phenomenological account with its concern for the proper 'foundations' for our understanding of medicine. This is most evident in the prevalence of classical (modern) foundationalist epistemologies in these discussions.[1] As part of the broader Enlightenment project of seeking to establish grounds for political engagement and scientific progress in forms of public discourse unsullied by vestiges of religion and other contentious traditions, classical foundationalism attempted to attain value-neutral, incorrigible bodies of knowledge that would be accepted by all rational agents – incorrigible and universally acceptable because they are neither subject to (the need for) correction nor open to (reasonable) doubt. That is to say, its aim was to strip away all the particularities of our experiences, the cultural frameworks that inform our beliefs, and the prejudices that affect our ability to see the way the world is in order to attain an objective viewpoint. Any belief or value not accepted by others in the conversation needed to be defended at the bar of reason; disagreement was evidence that someone had gone wrong somewhere in the formation of their beliefs. The proper exercise of reason would only allow beliefs and arguments that all reasonable people could rightly accept, with the result that all reasonable people would then necessarily agree with the conclusions. Values, traditions and (particularly) religious beliefs clearly get in the way of this, and so must be excluded from public rational discourse. Building on foundational beliefs of which we can be rightly certain, using methods that transfer that certitude to higher level beliefs, will result in bodies of knowledge that are both certain and not subject to correction. While there was entrenched disagreement about what counted as appropriate foundational beliefs and how such certainty might be transferred to the developed body of knowledge, something like this picture of how we ought to govern our beliefs has profoundly shaped the way we understand both science and public discourse. Unfortunately, this picture is profoundly mistaken.

First, it is fairly clear that science, the very model of modern rationality, is not conducted along (classical) foundationalist lines, and all attempts to (re)

[1] The following section draws upon my work in Andrew Sloane, *On Being a Christian in the Academy: Nicholas Wolterstorff and the Practice of Christian Scholarship* (Carlisle: Paternoster, 2003), and the literature cited therein, and on Nicholas Wolterstorff, *Reason within the Bounds of Religion*, 2nd edn. (Grand Rapids: Eerdmans, 1984) and *Until Justice and Peace Embrace* (Grand Rapids: Eerdmans, 1983).

construct it in conformity with this model of rationality have failed. Recent analyses of science and key moments in its development, have demonstrated that it does not operate according to any recognizable foundationalist patterns of rationality. Certainly, it does not operate by reasoning from indubitable foundations of 'objective' evidence by way of methods that transfer that indubitable status to higher order theories or beliefs. Indeed, much of the evidence used in classical scientific reasoning is 'theory-dependent', and many of the reasons on which theories are 'based' require tacit knowledge and non-rational modes of thought. This undermines classical modernist approaches to rationality (a fact that does not seem to have had the impact on some schools of thought in medicine that it ought to have had).

Second, the model is conceptually unsound, and in such a way that reconstruction of it is impossible. There is no means of connecting theories or higher-level beliefs with their foundations so as to transfer certitude from the foundations to the theories. Deduction, induction, falsificationism, abduction, and so on, may have legitimate roles to play in human reasoning; they do not, however, provide the objective, value-neutral certainty that foundationalism and the Enlightenment project demand. Even if they did, there is no foundation of certitudes upon which theories can be based. Sustained attempts to find such certainty in empirical observation and the clear distinction between observation statements and logically necessary beliefs (most importantly in the movement that became known as logical positivism or logical empiricism) failed. The reality of what has been called 'the theory dependence of observation statements' and the inability to demonstrate that what we think we experience is definitively grounded in reality, undercuts any claim to certainty in even the simplest observations of the world. In light of this, the value-neutral, consensus, absolutist notions of reason and scientific discourse associated with classical foundationalism are bankrupt.

In response to this, some have effectively surrendered either the notion that rationality is to guide our political or scientific discussions or the idea that 'truth' is the goal of our attempts to understand the world. There is no such thing as 'the way the world is' and even if there were, it is closed off to us by the ways we have been shaped by culture, language, tradition and beliefs. The idea seems to be that the only alternatives available to us are absolutist objectivity or irreducibly subjective relativism. This is, of course, a false antithesis;

nonetheless, such relativist or radically pluralist views have influenced some discussions of medicine and its practice.[2] Some lines of discussion depend on the idea that all our views of the world are governed by paradigms of knowing or worldviews, and that they are 'radically incommensurable'. That is, the language, ways of arguing, even ways of seeing the world that we depend on in our attempts to understand the world are *controlled* by the frameworks with which we operate (knowingly or unknowingly); we cannot step outside our framework of beliefs so as to see 'the way the world is'. Furthermore, people operating out of different frameworks see the world in such different ways that there is no real possibility of rational discussion across the borders of these conceptual countries and no way of adjudicating between the rival versions of the world constructed by them. This, too, is an unhelpful and misleading way of thinking about how we think about the world.

First, the claims such views make both about how we see the world and the ways in which disagreements between rival views of the world are conducted are unsound. Conceptual frameworks (often called paradigms or worldviews, unhelpfully in my view) are neither the monolithic entities nor as impermeable to critique as they are frequently presented as being. While claims made in one systemic context cannot simply be transferred to another, it is possible to communicate across the borders of conceptual systems in much the same way that translation is possible between languages. Something is always lost in translation, but communication is possible and, given care, it is possible to engage in reasoned argument. There is no guarantee, of course, that such discussion will end in agreement; but then, debate is the lifeblood of the academy and need not be seen as a failure of one party or another to properly engage in it. Second, there is, in fact, no way of coherently asserting relativism or radical pluralism or ideological reconstructions of scientific knowledge. If all knowledge is relative or radically plural so that there is no 'true' way of seeing the world, only different perspectives on it, then how is it that such a statement can be meaningfully made? If all knowledge claims are disguised grabs for power, then so is this claim. For these 'radical theories' are making a

2 See, for instance, Kazem Sadegh-Zadeh, The Logic of Diagnosis, in *Philosophy of Medicine*, ed. Fred Gifford (Amsterdam: Elsevier, 2011) and his claim that diagnoses in medicine are 'social acts that create social facts' (358).

claim about reality (the reality of human knowledge rather than other features of the world, admittedly, but reality nonetheless); either their claims are true, in which case they are relative, or radically pluralist, or disguised acts of power, and so do not give us a true picture of the nature of human knowing; or they do give us a true picture of how we know the world, in which case those claims are not radically relative, or pluralist, or acts of social control, and so they are false. The only escape from the horns of this logical dilemma is either to excuse those claims from their own force (and what reason could we have to do that?) or to accept that such claims fail by virtue of 'self-referential incoherence': which is to say, they cannot be asserted without undermining themselves or falling prey to incoherence.

That is not to say that we can somehow stand outside the intellectual frameworks, traditions and perspectives that shape our beliefs and ways of seeing the world; nor is it to say that we are somehow morally pristine knowers such that our belief-formation is quarantined from our interests and ideologies and the systems of power and control in which we are enmeshed. All knowledge is partial, all beliefs subject to correction, all perspectives distorted by where we find ourselves in the world, at times culpably so, and this impinges on our ability to access reality. In this respect at least, 'postmodern' philosophy and critical theory need to be factored into our epistemologies – including our understanding of medicine and medical knowing. Nonetheless, given the implausibility of the alternatives, the way is clear for a defeasible, situation- and person-specific understanding of rationality and public discourse. And, indeed, there are good theological reasons for developing such a view. For none of us have a 'God's-eye view' of the world; we are all finite and limited in our knowledge of it; further, sin has such deep roots in the fabric of our being, including our reason, that our beliefs and the ways we form them are distorted by self-interest, false values, oppressive social and intellectual traditions, and so on; even so, we have been made by God in such a way that we do have real access to the world – partial and flawed, but real.[3] However, for such an epistemology to work, we need to reconsider both the status of our beliefs and the structure of our belief systems.

3 I will explore this in some detail below.

A key element of many epistemologies is what has been called a 'guilty-until-proven-innocent' view of rationality. What this means is that beliefs are only considered reasonable if we have (demonstrable) reason to accept or maintain them. In relation to our beliefs, absence of evidence (or reasons) is evidence of absence of rationality, for it demonstrates a failure in our governing of our beliefs and belief-formation. Such an epistemology is implicit (and frequently explicit) in the evidence-based medicine movement: the very term indicates both its foundationalism (evidence-*based* medicine) and its commitment to the requirement that beliefs need to prove themselves before we are entitled to accept (and act upon) them (*evidence*-based medicine). On the surface, that seems reasonable and rigorously 'scientific'; unfortunately, it is neither. Not only is it not 'scientific', at least in the sense of how (good) science actually operates, neither is it reasonable. For many, indeed most, of our most important beliefs are neither held on the basis of sufficient evidence nor would they pass such a test were it applied to them. Our knowledge of other persons, their interests, desires, personality, and so on, and even basic beliefs about the world, do not work that way.

The beliefs about the world that we form using our perceptual apparatus cannot pass the 'guilty-until-proven-innocent' test: for such beliefs, and any 'evidence' we might use to support them, use the very perceptual system that is under question. But equally, the way our beliefs are actually formed fits neither the 'guilty-until-proven-innocent' criterion, nor the pattern of belief-formation by way of inference from observation. We do not look out the window and by a series of inferences come to the conclusion that we see a tree waving in the breeze on a sunny day because this has been demonstrated to be the case by the evidence of our senses. These are beliefs that are formed in us using, say, vision; but they are not formed by way of inferences from perceptual experiences. Rather, in looking out the window we see the tree *as* a tree waving in the breeze on a sunny day and we come to believe, not primarily that we *see* the tree, but that the tree is there, really waving in the breeze on a sunny day in the actual world. This may seem obvious, but it has important implications for how we think about thinking, and how we reason about reason. In particular, these observations (and myriad others) render implausible the basic picture of how beliefs work that we've taken for granted: for beliefs need to be seen not as the result of a process of inference (from evidence) which need to be shown to be sound before we're entitled to believe them, but as the result of 'belief-forming mechanisms' or 'practices of inquiry'. Furthermore, we are entitled to accept these beliefs unless something can be shown to have gone wrong in their formation, especially in the way we have conducted ourselves as epistemic agents (that is, as those direct our affairs, including observations, reason, and so on, in order to make sense of the world).

This alternative understanding radically changes the nature of 'pre-understanding', or the 'cloak of beliefs' we all find ourselves with. While our presuppositions need to be critically scrutinized for their reliability, they are not an irrational impediment to a proper understanding of the world, but contribute to that understanding (and necessarily so). Even the most basic of our beliefs come to us already 'loaded' conceptually. Seeing a tree waving in the breeze on a sunny day presupposes beliefs and assumptions about trees, wind, sunshine, and even the basically non-distorting transparency of glass. We may not be aware of those presuppositions; indeed, we generally are not focally aware of them. Rather, they form part of the cloak of beliefs with which we are clothed; none of us engages the world as naked epistemic agents. If we were to do so, we would not get very far in our attempts to understand the world. Even what we take as straightforward observations about the world come so clothed. This is, I think, particularly clear in the case of medical knowledge. Much of what we 'see' or 'feel' in medicine depends on deep and complex theoretical structures. Palpation of an abdomen only gives us meaningful knowledge if we have a basic understanding of human anatomy and so an expectation of what we ought to feel where and what it ought to feel like. That knowledge allows us to feel granular hepatomegaly and, indeed, to feel an enlarged cirrhotic liver, but only after we have been inducted into the knowledge and skills we need in order to feel it. Viewing an X-ray presupposes basic knowledge of both anatomy and the relative radio-opacity of different tissues, and experience and skill in interpreting other X-rays. That knowledge allows us to see a fractured clavicle (or wonder whether we see a fractured scaphoid), but only after we have been inducted into the knowledge and skills we need in order to see it, and to know that what we see on a viewing box or monitor corresponds in some way to what is going on in a patient's body. Basic medical observations come cloaked with a complex set of beliefs without which we would not have the knowledge that informs clinical judgement and which, in turn, enables good clinical decision making.

Furthermore, we function as *agents* in our knowing. Most epistemologies have been both overly passive and inadequately embodied. They see us as passive receivers of information on which we go to work with our minds. But that is not generally how we do things. Rather, we are active: we look out the window to see what it's like outside; we look up the normal range of serum Creatinine; we ask a colleague whether they see hairline fracture or not. And our knowledge has history, it is embedded in a community and in traditions of knowledge and skill of which we are both heirs and custodians. Our knowledge is active, traditioned and communal. Moreover, we are knowing bodies: our physical apparatus enables us to see and hear and touch, and even to go down the hall to ask a colleague their opinion.

While these beliefs and traditions of knowing enable us to get in touch with the world, they also both limit and distort our knowledge of it. They shape what things and kinds of things we look for and how we look for them, and so limit what we see and what kinds of things we can see. We may 'see' things that are not there (the 'disease of masturbation', for instance, in Engelhardt's famous piece[4]); we may not see things that are there, even refuse to see them (chronic fatigue syndrome (CFS) in the late twentieth century). Much of that is simply the consequence of where we find ourselves in human history; we are wrong about the world, but we have done no wrong in our attempts to understand and engage in it. Doctors who ascribed malaria to 'bad air' were wrong, but in the absence of complex germ theories of disease, knowledge of parasitology, vectors, and so forth, their failure to ascribe it to the malaria parasite and to recognize the Anopheles mosquito as the primary mode of transmission was not due to a failure on their part as knowing agents. But some of that false perception, some of those erroneous claims to knowledge, may be linked to culpable failures in our conduct as knowing agents, even systemic flaws in the systems that have shaped us. The belief that sufferers from CFS were malingering was the result both of an inability to detect subtle changes in the immune system and overly positivist understandings of medicine. The absence of demonstrable pathology on laboratory tests led doctors to conclude that there was nothing wrong with these patients.

[4] H. Tristram Engelhardt, Jr, The Disease of Masturbation: Values and the Concept of Disease, in *Meaning and Medicine: A Reader in the Philosophy of Health Care*, ed. H. L. Nelson and J. L. Nelson (New York: Routledge, 1999).

This means that, while our beliefs may be 'innocent-until-proven-guilty', they are not quarantined from critical appraisal, and nor are the assumptions and systems of knowledge that give rise to them. There is an apparent tension here. We need not 'prove' our beliefs before we are entitled to accept them, nor is it possible to subject them to that kind of criticism; unless we have good reason to think otherwise, we are entitled to hold the beliefs we have. However, our beliefs do need to be subject to critical scrutiny, for we miss some things and get other things wrong. The way to resolve this tension is relatively easy, so long as we free ourselves from the irrational constraints of modernist epistemology. We need to understand rationality as person- and situation-specific and as defeasible. That is to say, what is reasonable for a person to believe, what is appropriate for them to believe, depends on who they are, their background and context. Rationality, however, needs to be carefully distinguished from truth. Our aim is to come to grips with the truth, with the way things are; but we need to recognize that our grip on reality is partial and flawed, and so our beliefs need to be subject to correction. They are defeasible. We come to see that when something goes wrong in our beliefs: there's something missing in our view of the world; we were wrong in what we thought was going on; we come to the painful realization that our beliefs and the systems that gave rise to them have been distorted by self-interest and wrongful exercise of power. And we try to figure out what went wrong in our beliefs and how we can go about fixing it.

Nicholas Wolterstorff's epistemology

Let me turn for a moment to an attempt to frame this more systematically, drawing on the work of Nicholas Wolterstorff.[5] Central to Wolterstorff's understanding are the notions that our beliefs are the product of belief-dispositions (or belief-forming mechanisms, such as perception, memory, introspection, and so on) or practices of inquiry (which involves the use of belief-forming mechanisms in particular goal-oriented projects), and that they are, in general, innocent-until-proven-guilty (as explored above). In light of this, his concept of entitlement to beliefs focuses on the removal of justification

5 See Sloane, *On Being a Christian in the Academy*, Part Three.

or entitlement from a particular person's acceptance of particular beliefs, and on the proper governance of practices of inquiry so as to get in touch with reality. One crucial cause of distortion in believing and a paradigm case of what counts against the accepting or holding onto particular beliefs is 'the noetic effects of sin'. That is to say, sin influences not just the motives we have for forming particular beliefs or the goals towards which we direct our projects, it corrupts reason itself and our use of it, as well as the traditions into which we are inducted and which shape our understanding of the world and how we consider we ought to go about understanding it.

Wolterstorff's understanding of reason is both situated and non-absolutist, since a particular person's obligations in relation to the conduct of their quest to understand the world depend upon their particular context, and indeed are a function of their general obligations. Wolterstorff sees being reasonable as a matter of fulfilling those obligations that rightly have bearing on our belief-formation. Those obligations are not, however, a matter of *choosing* to believe such-and-such; our beliefs are not the product of our choices, but of those mechanisms that form beliefs in us. Our obligations, then, relate to the governing of our use of our belief-forming apparatus so as to get in touch with reality. However, those obligations are limited, for having right beliefs about the world is not the only thing that matters to us, or to the communities of which we are a part, or to the God whom we serve. Indeed, our obligations in relation to our beliefs (call them *noetic obligations*) arise in and are justified by circumstances in which we find ourselves and the tasks to which we are called. So too, they only entail that we do as well as can be rightly expected of us to avoid error and attain truth, not that we actually do so. Nonetheless, his is a rational epistemology, for he believes that we are constrained by the natures of reality and of God so as to make the quest for truth possible and necessary.

Wolterstorff's associated understanding of scholarly practice is a product of the Dutch Neo-Calvinist tradition, but he departs from it in important respects. One key problem with many Calvinist understandings of scholarship is their notion that, because Christians and non-Christians start from different premises and operate according to different rules, they will produce radically different bodies of knowledge. Thus, there are 'Two Sciences', Christian and non-Christian, for non-Christian scholarship inevitably falls prey to the reductionism of idolatry, and so at crucial points Christian scholars must necessarily part company from their non-Christian colleagues. Important conceptual and empirical problems with these claims gave rise to and also justify Wolterstorff's rejection of their views; nonetheless, he embraced important elements of the Neo-Calvinist rejection of autonomous, religiously neutral scholarship. The most important difference between his and earlier Reformed theories of science is his claim that a Christian scholar is called to be *faithful* rather than *different* in their scholarly practice. The way this is fleshed out in his understanding of scholarship depends upon his understanding of the role of beliefs and commitments in the devising and weighing of theories. He distinguished between *data beliefs* (beliefs we form about what we take to be facts of the matter), *data-background beliefs* (those beliefs that shape what we count as data or facts of the matter and how we go about finding out about them) and *control beliefs*. While the differences between these beliefs are differences of function rather than of kind, the nature and role of control beliefs lie at the heart of his understanding of the practice of Christian scholarship.

Wolterstorff presents control beliefs as those of our beliefs that prompt us to accept or reject theories and to devise the sorts of theories that we do: they are, as the term suggests, beliefs that have a controlling, or gate-keeping function in our belief systems. Crucial to his understanding of scholarship, and what makes scholarship *Christian* is the way that 'the belief-content of authentic Christian commitment' ought to function as a control in a Christian scholar's devising and weighing of theories. Authentic Christian commitment is a selection from among the obligations that a Christian scholar has: it is person- and situation-specific, as is its belief content. It operates as a control by means of the governing of our doxastic practices (that is, how we use our belief-forming mechanisms) so as to accept and devise complex sets of beliefs and reject others. However, the interaction between the belief content of authentic Christian commitment and particular bodies of knowledge is complex: at times a body of knowledge will alter what a Christian scholar takes to be the belief content of their authentic Christian commitment;[6] at others, a

6 For instance, the recognition that Scripture does not require a geocentric cosmology. It must be noted that the history of the shift from a dominant geocentric cosmology to and beyond heliocentric ones is much more complex than popular histories of science suggest, and resistance to the shift owed more to internal ecclesial politics and the dominance of Aristotelian physics and metaphysics than to the Church's resistance to science.

theory may give way before it.[7] Which of these happens on a given occasion depends upon person- and situation-specific factors, and should do so. For these, and other reasons, there is no 'algorithm of rationality', no fixed and deterministic set of procedures that when undertaken guarantee rational belief (let alone the truth). The quest for truth is, however, the goal of our theoretical practices, at least in as much as this relates to our governing of which beliefs or theories we ought to accept.

Things are a little more complicated in the area of *heuristics*, that is, the decisions we make about what research projects or intellectual enterprises we should engage in. It is commonly held that selecting a particular research agenda ought also to be governed by the quest for truth; that, in Wolterstorff's view, is a mistake. The quest for truth is, he believes, the domain of what he calls acceptance-governance (that is, the decisions we make about how we govern our practices of inquiry so as to accept certain beliefs or theories and reject others). Instead heuristics, the decisions a scholar makes about which research tradition they ought to pursue, is to be governed by the quest for *shalom*. Wolterstorff believes that justice-in-*shalom* is the ultimate *telos* of human life.[8] The primary obligation of Christians is to foster the quest for justice-in-*shalom*, and so it should govern both the decisions they make about the course their life should take and, for those who embrace a call to the academy, also their scholarly practice. Knowledge is itself an aspect of *shalom*, and can also contribute to the quest for liberation. Thus the heuristics of *shalom* warrants both pure theory, which aims simply at understanding the world and how it operates without explicitly considering its benefits for people and the world, as well as (more obviously) praxis-oriented theory, which aims at generating knowledge for the benefit of humanity and the world in which we live. Which particular research tradition a scholar pursues is a context-specific decision. Such decisions, Wolterstorff contends, must take account of the operation of sinful doxastic practices, which give rise to and sustain research traditions that foster the selfish agenda of individuals or powerful

7 For instance, strict behaviourist (or other reductionist) psychological theories.

8 It is important to note how this differs from classical Thomistic notions of the beatific vision which generates significant tensions for Christian understanding of and engaging in the world (including medicine), as I noted in Chapter 6 in relation to Messer's work on health.

elites. Christian scholars should faithfully and openly listen to the Word of God and the cries of the oppressed in order to unmask the operation of these sinful vested interests. This notion of the heuristics of *shalom* plays an important role, I would suggest, in Christian understandings of medicine and how it ought to operate. In particular, it allows us to address systematically and faithfully the legitimate concerns raised about the ways in which medical research (and practice) generally focuses on 'first world problems' rather than those of the majority world, often in order to foster the vested interests and even the idolatrous delusions of powerful elites in wealthier communities.

Epistemology and theories of medicine

I will return to some of these matters later, when I look at the form of medical knowing and how we should think about it as Christians. For now, my chief concern is to demonstrate that Christians are entitled to allow their understanding of their Christian faith to impact on their understanding of and engagement in their intellectual pursuits; they are, in fact, required to do so.[9] The results may or may not differ in important ways from the work of their non-Christian colleagues. They need not do so as a matter of principle: the principle at stake is whether a Christian is true to their Christian commitment, not whether that cashes out in different ways to their colleagues' practice. Again: Christians are called to be *faithful* not just *different*. However, it is very likely that such faithful scholarly engagement may differ from non-Christian scholarship, and for a number of reasons.[10] One is the notion of the 'heart', so beloved of strands of Calvinist (and Augustinian) theology. The 'heart' speaks of our fundamental orientation, the beliefs, practices and passions that govern our lives and direct them towards or away from God and God's kingly purposes in the world.[11] All

9 For a recent attempt to do so, see Allen Verhey, Can Calvin Save Medicine? A Response to Jeff Bishop, *Christian Bioethics* 20, no. 1 (2014).

10 And, for that matter, engagement in the 'real world' – as if scholarship isn't a real-world enterprise. But I must leave those questions to one side.

11 James K. A. Smith, *Desiring the Kingdom: Worship, Worldview, and Cultural Formation* (Grand Rapids: Eerdmans, 2009) has rightly criticized 'worldview' approaches for their overly cognitive view of human beliefs and behaviour, and emphasized the importance of both the affections and the nature of bodily existence in shaping human life and faith.

of our hearts are marred by sin such that our loves are not 'true' (in the sense of lining up the way they should; they are out of kilter), and so neither are our lives. However, a Christian's heart is (or ought to be) being reshaped by the agency of the Spirit so as to orient and reorient it towards God and God's transformative purposes in Christ. Thus there is (or should be) a fundamental difference between the hearts of Christians and non-Christians, and so the direction their lives take, including those aspects of life related to their beliefs and professional practice. In many respects, those beliefs and practices relate to matters fairly distant from the 'heart' of the matter. They deal with matters that do not impinge greatly on our fundamental orientation and the passions and practices that govern our lives. For instance, particular biochemical or physiological theories are unlikely to bring our fundamental orientation into play; there is little reason to expect that a Christian biochemist will come up with a different understanding of intracellular metabolism than their non-Christian colleague. Seeking to understand human sexuality, however, or the nature and goals of key institutions and their role in society, is very likely to bring the heart into play, as they deal with things that matter deeply to us, and the beliefs and values that govern our lives. Given the nature of medicine and the way it deals with fundamental features of the human condition and as a practice is deeply imbued with (moral) values, it is reasonable to expect that a Christian understanding of medicine will take a different shape to other ways of thinking about it. The nature of Christian commitment and the way it shapes our beliefs, values, passions and practices will give rise to a particular way of understanding medicine and its goals. But in order to be clear about that, we first need to be clear about what we believe as Christians and how that might affect our understanding both of epistemology and of medicine.

A theological framework: biblical theology and God's story

Understanding scholarship in light of (the propositional content of) Christian faith requires some understanding of what that faith looks like. Of course, Scripture says little directly about medicine, or epistemology for that matter; it certainly has no 'theory' of medicine or epistemology that we can mine from its pages. But that is beside the point; for my claim is not that Christian scholars or doctors ought to conform their practice to the direct dictates of Scripture, but that the key beliefs that shape Christian commitment and which arise, in turn, from Scripture are to function as a control on their practice. Still, some particular construal of that faith will govern the enterprise. While there are many contenders, I take a narratively driven biblical theology as my starting point, in part because of its inherent strengths, and in part because it provides a helpful set of lenses through which to view both scholarship in general and medicine in particular. The narrative helps us to understand both our location in God's kingly purposes and some of the tensions and puzzles that beset understanding what medicine is and is about.[12]

The very possibility of biblical theology has come under attack in recent scholarship from a number of points of view. James Barr has argued that the programme was infected from the start with false contrasts between 'Hebrew' and 'Greek' thought forms, and mistaken linguistic and theological claims.[13] Classical historical-critics argue that the biblical literature is too diverse, even contradictory in its claims to be synthesized in a coherent biblical theology. Biblical *theology* is impossible, we can only develop biblical *theologies*, or better, theologies of different books, authors, corpora or traditions.[14] Further, the major exemplars of the programme, such as the magisterial theologies of Eichrodt and von Rad in the Old Testament, or Bultmann in the New, have been (rightly in my view) rejected as procrustean.[15] Postmodern theologians and biblical scholars such as Walter Brueggemann have suggested that the task

[12] A biblical-theological framework for understanding biomedical ethics is the burden of James Rusthoven, *Covenantal Biomedical Ethics for Contemporary Medicine: An Alternative to Principles-Based Ethics* (Eugene, OR: Pickwick, 2014), esp. Part Two. Unfortunately, he is too dependent on *covenant* as a dominant organizing principle in biblical theology and on Dooyeweerd's worldview-driven approach to Christian philosophy. I will demonstrate below that, while useful, covenant is not an adequate construal of biblical-theology. For a brief critique of Dooyeweerd's version of Reformed philosophy, see Sloane, *On Being a Christian in the Academy*, 118–126.

[13] James Barr, *The Semantics of Biblical Language* (Oxford: Oxford University Press, 1961). It should be noted, however, that he has moderated his claims in his later work, noting that his critiques were directed towards the 'biblical-theology' movement, not the notion of biblical theology *per se*, for which see *The Concept of Biblical Theology: An Old Testament Perspective* (London: SCM, 1999), esp. 146–171.

[14] Petr Pokorny, The Problem of Biblical Theology, *Horizons in Biblical Theology* 15, no. 1 (1993); Heikki Räisänen, *Beyond New Testament Theology: A Story and a Programme* (London: SCM, 1990), esp. xv–xviii, 117–118.

[15] See the essays in Steven J. Kraftchick, Jr, Charles D. Myers, and Ben C. Ollenburger (eds.), *Biblical Theology: Problems and Perspectives* (Nashville: Abingdon, 1995).

founders on a multiplicity of pluralities: of theologies within Scripture (or *testimonies* to use Brueggemann's terminology); interpretive methods that can be applied to the texts; and interpretive communities.[16] It seems that the obstacles in my path are insuperable.

But perhaps not. First, these claims are all strongly contested in biblical theology.[17] Second, most of them fall shy of the mark in relation to *my* construal of biblical theology, in which narrative plays a constitutive role.[18] Crucial to my understanding of biblical theology is the notion of *story*, for when Christians (and Jews for that matter) are asked to give an account of the hope that is in them they will generally tell a story. That story goes something like this.

The story begins with God, the triune God who exists in relationship as Father, Son and Spirit (Genesis 1, John 1). God created the cosmos and all that is in it in a manner that reflects God's own character, including the very fact of order and the fundamentally relational character of existence. This creation was good – it worked the way God intended it to work. As part of this creation, and as those given responsibility over some of its governance, God created human beings. God created humans in the image and likeness of God, in a particular pattern of relationship with God, each other and the world. From the beginning, then, humans are social beings, and embodied beings who inhabit God's world as God's people (Gen 1:26–28, 2:7, 18–25). Each of these points has important implications for Christian epistemology, for the character of God's creative and providential action, and the embodied nature of human existence, ground the very possibility of human knowledge, as well as its nature and limitations. Furthermore, the knowledge that this is a world created in sovereign

16 Walter Brueggemann, Biblical Theology Appropriately Postmodern, *Biblical Theology Bulletin* 27 (1997); *Theology of the Old Testament: Testimony, Dispute, Advocacy* (Minneapolis: Fortress, 1997), esp. xv–xvii, 71–84.

17 Bernhard W. Anderson and Steven Bishop, *Contours of Old Testament Theology* (Minneapolis: Fortress, 1998); Don Carson, Current Issues in Biblical Theology: A New Testament Perspective, *Bulletin for Biblical Research* 5 (1995).

18 For articulations and defences of a narrative approach to (biblical) theology, see Craig G. Bartholomew and Michael W. Goheen, *The Drama of Scripture: Finding Our Place in the Biblical Story* (Grand Rapids: Baker Academic, 2004); Stephen G. Dempster, *Dominion and Dynasty: A Theology of the Hebrew Bible* (Leicester: Apollos, 2003); Gabriel Fackre, *The Christian Story*, 3rd edn. (Grand Rapids: Eerdmans, 1996); George Lindbeck, *The Nature of Doctrine: Religion and Theology in a Postliberal Age* (Philadelphia: Westminster, 1984), esp. 112–138; C. Marvin Pate et al., *The Story of Israel: A Biblical Theology* (Leicester: Apollos, 2004); Thomas R. Schreiner, *The King in His Beauty: A Biblical Theology of the Old and New Testaments* (Grand Rapids: Baker, 2013); Christopher J. H. Wright, *The Mission of God: Unlocking the Bible's Grand Narrative* (Nottingham: IVP, 2006).

freedom by God means that if we are to understand it we need to 'look and see' what God has done. It also has bearing on our understanding of medicine and the way that care for embodied creatures coheres with our created nature and, indeed, on the importance of seeking to understand how we operate.

Human beings are created in the image of God and given dominion over creation. This legitimates the human quest for knowledge and our actions in the world which aim to bring creation into line with God's purposes. We are made in the image of God, with the corresponding responsibility to live rightly before God, with each other and in the world, including the exercise of loving dominion in it. The quest for understanding is both good in its own right and also serves the end of our service of God, each other and the creation, including the responsibility to be agents of God's ordering purposes in the world. This is complicated in relation to medical research and practice, for we are not only those who look at and act in the world, we are also that which is examined and acted upon. We can, then, legitimately turn our scrutiny on ourselves and our biological and psychological systems and seek to ensure their proper functioning. Nonetheless, we are still creatures, kin with creation – and there is an objective order to the world and ourselves. Thus, there are limits to what we can and should do in both research and practice, ensuring we neither violate the integrity of creation, nor overstep the bounds of creaturely responsibility. So, views of science and technology – including medical science and medical technology – that see it as freeing us from all human limitation fail to reckon with the givenness of the human created condition.

However, as we are all too aware, the world we inhabit is 'not the way it's supposed to be' – and nor are we.[19] For sin entered the picture (Genesis 3). Whatever the 'origins of evil', humanity used its God-given freedom-in-responsibility, including the freedom of interpersonal relationships, in a manner contrary to God's good purposes. Sin now distorts relationships between humans and God, each other and the world, and even the way in which the world works.[20]

19 Cornelius Plantinga, *Not the Way It's Supposed to Be: A Breviary of Sin* (Grand Rapids: Eerdmans, 1995).

20 The question of whether human sin has direct effects on the physical world or whether it distorts creation only indirectly, by way of humanity's failure to govern it aright, and by way of humanity's sinful abuse of it, is not germane to my argument. For my purposes, all that matters is that sin *does* distort the world and, more particularly, our interaction with it and other persons: the mechanism is irrelevant.

This, too, has important epistemological implications, in as much as it explains the fractured and flawed nature of our knowledge of the world, the way in which our relationships and intellectual communities can frustrate as well as foster truthful engagement with the world, and the fact that we tend to suppress, avoid, misuse and distort the truth to further our own ends.

The fallenness of creation, including human creatures, clearly warrants medical research and practice, as is almost universally acknowledged. It is not only the world in which we live that is 'not the way it's supposed to be'; so are our bodies and psyches. It is not just creation that groans, so do we. But that brokenness is complicated, including as it does both pathology and the orderly responses of the body to it. We need to understand the normal operation of ourselves as biological and psychological systems, how pathogens and other noxious environmental phenomena operate on their own terms, as well as how they interact with us and our functioning and how we respond to them. This, as all medical students know, is a complex matter, requiring knowledge, insight and skill in order to both understand what might be going wrong and then figure out what to do about it. Furthermore, this fallen world is characterized by disadvantage and the misuse of power. Our calling is to use the knowledge and power entrusted to us in service of those who most need it, very often those who are disadvantaged by the very systems that give us the freedom to embrace that calling. But we must do so in the awareness that we and others have an inherent tendency to use our knowledge and power for our own interests and the interests of those like us who benefit from the distorted systems in which we find ourselves. Thus we need to challenge both medical technology and its uses to determine whether it is a faithful exploration of God's creation, and beneficial for God's creatures, including ourselves. We need to ask the old Latin judicial question: 'Who benefits?' Will this research benefit all humanity or just a privileged few? Does this treatment option open up freedom for all, or does it advantage those who already benefit from life's lottery? Even so, this world while fallen is still God's creation, as are we. We need to think carefully about how what we do lines up with or against God's creational purposes, whether it abets the corrupting power of sin or combats it and its effects.

The God who made the cosmos and humanity did so with certain purposes, or ends, in mind; and God will not allow these purposes to be finally frustrated.

So God 'enters into' human affairs in judgement and grace in order to bring these ends to pass. Central to this story in the Old Testament is the election of Abraham, and so of the nation Israel (Genesis 12; Exodus 19:4–6). By this choice, God's saving acts of power, and particularly the covenant God makes with Israel, God brings into being a new community that is meant to reflect the character of God and God's rule, and so live in a manner coordinate with God's creative purposes. Israel's history, however, demonstrates their failure to 'live as the people of God', despite God's acts of grace and judgement in Israel's history.[21]

Once more, God's purposes will not be thwarted, so God acts in a radically new way in the incarnation and ministry of the Son, Jesus Christ. The history of God and the world finds its goal in the life and ministry of Jesus the Messiah (John 1; Ephesians 1; Hebrews 1:1–4). In the gospels, we see the Son of God 'enfleshed', dwelling bodily among us. He is true God and true human, and so reveals to us the character of God, of ideal humanity, and of God's pattern of relationships. He is the embodiment of the truth of *shalom* (e.g., John 14:6). Through his death and resurrection, he pays the penalty for Israel and so for us, and inaugurates the eschatological restoration of relationships with God, each other and the created order (Romans 1–8; Colossians 1; Hebrews 2, 8–10; 1 John 1:5–2:2).[22] This, too, is important for Christian epistemology and for compassionate action in the world, as it tells us that we are not trapped in blindness and error and selfishness and injustice. For the God who made us, among other things to know God, each other and the world, has acted to do what we could not do, and rescue us from the hopeless systematic distortion of our cognitive faculties and to give us new freedom by the Spirit to act as agents of God's purposes in the world. This, however, needs to be understood in light of the final stage of the story, lest we be too triumphalistic in our assessment of our 'noetic redemption' or our moral capacities.

The end of this history is a new beginning in which God's purposes for humanity and the world are achieved – purposes which seem to transcend or surpass those of the original state (Revelation 21-22). In this final state, the

21 Following Christopher J. H. Wright, *Old Testament Ethics for the People of God* (Leicester: IVP, 2004).

22 Andrew Sloane, Justice and the Atonement in the Book of Isaiah, *Trinity Journal* 34NS, no. 1 (2013).

cosmos itself will be transformed, and so will we (Romans 8). Sin will no longer be a factor in human existence; we will know fully and we will know truly.[23] A number of things are important to note about the *eschaton*. First, it is a future that awaits us; second, it has become a force in human history, by way of God's gracious action in Jesus and the work of the Holy Spirit; third, an important mark, or component, of that action is a new community in which we are called to live out the (re)new(ed) pattern of relationships. We live, as has often been noted, in the tension of the 'now and not yet', and we do so as participants in a new community.[24] This, too, has an important role to play in the development of Christian epistemology. For it means, first, that the *truth* is a worthy goal; second, that it is a goal that we will never attain in history; but third, that it is worth striving for, since God is at work bringing the reality of the future of truth to bear on our present.

The thankful realization that God has acted in history to redeem us, particularly in the life, ministry, death and resurrection of Jesus and continues to be at work to renew us and creation, and has invited us to be his agents in his world has significant implications for medical research and practice. First, it grounds our searching for solutions to the problems we and vulnerable people face in the world, for God is at work restoring broken order and invites us to participate in that work, both as knowers and actors in this world which is still God's. Second, it places all we do in the broader context of the Kingdom of God, and our knowledge of what God's kingly rule looks like in light of Christ, and our anticipation of its final consummation in the *eschaton*. And so we need to ask how and in what ways do our research and practice conform or not to the character of the Kingdom of God; further, what priority do they have *vis-à-vis* other aspects of this Kingdom work, especially in light of God's well-known 'preferential option for the poor'? Indeed, in light of Deuteronomy (esp. Deut. 10:12–22) and Matthew 25, we need to recognize that care for the vulnerable is one of the key expressions of a properly formed human community, one that reflects the character of God and so is a necessary feature

[23] At least, we will know as fully and as truly as we are able to know as finite creatures, for I take it that sin, rather than creaturely finitude, will be overcome.

[24] Richard Hays, *The Moral Vision of the New Testament: A Contemporary Introduction to New Testament Ethics* (New York: HarperCollins, 1996). This is, of course, an important element in Hauerwas' theological understanding of (ethics and) medicine.

of those communities that claim to model themselves on the character of the creating, redeeming, transforming God of love. Moreover, as Luke 13:16 reminds us, the restoration of physical well-being is one sign of the sabbatical freedom of the Kingdom of God. We need to realize, however, that the full healing of humanity and final transformation of the world await the return of Jesus the King. In the meantime, we live 'between the times', looking for and working towards signs of God's kingly rule in the world, and longing for the return of Jesus. While he brought the restoration of relationships and creation order that characterizes the coming of the Kingdom of God, healing the sick, calming the storm, feeding the hungry, even raising the dead, this, too, is a foretaste of the future fullness. For the sick and raised became sick again and died, storms still rage, people still are hungry. So, once again, we live 'between the ages', knowing in part, awaiting full knowledge, recognizing that we have no technological saviour. Science and technology, and the therapies they give rise to, are good and useful but are no more than a means we use to do what we can to conform creation to the coming kingdom as we live between the ages. This, again, places clear limits on what we can and should do and provides an overarching conceptual schema for our understanding and practice of medicine.

However, above all, perhaps, biblical theology reminds us that we are fundamentally relational beings created for community; thus, our ability to function in meaningful relationships with God, each other and creation as a whole is our most basic capacity. That capacity, however, should not be seen as what gives us ontological and hence moral value.[25] Our inherent value is the product of God's creating and redeeming grace (Psalm 8; Rom. 14:1–15:13; 1 Cor. 8:9–13) which both constitutes us as beings of a particular kind and also (and thereby) grants us particular standing in relation to God, the world and other creatures and in our social relationships (Gen. 9:6). Nonetheless, the exercise of those relational capacities is fundamental to human agency, and the

[25] This is, of course, a complex and contentious matter that has received a great deal of attention, especially in relation to disputes over 'sanctity' and 'quality' of life as determinants of decisions regarding appropriate medical care and questions of the nature of 'personhood' as that which morally distinguishes humans from other creatures (or not). I believe a more fruitful line can be developed in relation to appropriate care, especially of the dying, which will be discussed in Chapter 9 below.

properly formed human community. The idea that best captures the nature of the properly formed human community is *shalom*, a rich and complex notion that plays an important role in biblical theology and Christian understanding of science, technology and other cultural expressions of human agency. 'Shalom is a picture of community, of life in relationships, in which things are as they are supposed to be. Humans live in harmony and delight with God, each other and the world. In *shalom*, people live lives characterized by love, justice and faithfulness.'[26] Understanding the nature of the flourishing which is *shalom* and seeking to enhance it is the goal of human knowledge; seeking to overcome that which might inhibit a person's ability to flourish and that of the physical and relational systems in which they find themselves is the goal of human agency. It is those capacities that enable us to function well in relationships that are the focus of care – including medical care – and establish the appropriate limits of it. As I will explore in the next two chapters, this has implications for the nature and limits of our care.

Mark 5:25-34 – a case in point

Having outlined a biblical-theological framework for understanding medicine, I think it's worth our while pausing to reflect on a paradigmatic story: Jesus' healing of the woman with menorrhagia. I will take the version of the story found in Mark's gospel (Mk. 5:25–34), in part because it is the fullest of the synoptic accounts, in part because it includes what Luke doesn't – the detail of the powerlessness of the medicine of the day to deal with her condition (perhaps, an indication of the close connection between the 'beloved physician' and the gospel?).[27]

[26] Andrew Sloane, *At Home in a Strange Land: Using the Old Testament in Christian Ethics* (Peabody/Grand Rapids: Hendrickson/Baker, 2008), 28, drawing on the excellent, brief articulation of *shalom* in Wolterstorff, *Until Justice and Peace Embrace*, 69–72.

[27] For helpful exegetical observations on the text, see Mary Ann Beavis, *Mark* (Grand Rapids: Baker, 2011), 95–98; C. Clifton Black, *Mark* (Nashville: Abingdon, 2011), 139–145; R. Alan Cole, *Mark: An Introduction and Commentary* (Nottingham: IVP, 1989), 163–169; John R. Donahue and Daniel J. Harrington, *The Gospel of Mark* (Collegeville: Liturgical Press, 2002), 171–182; R. T. France, *The Gospel of Mark: A Commentary on the Greek Text* (Grand Rapids: Eerdmans, 2002), 233–240; Robert A. Guelich, *Mark 1-8:26* (Dallas: Word, 1989), 289–305; Larry W. Hurtado, *Mark* (Peabody: Hendrickson, 1989), 86–92; Donald H. Juel, *Mark* (Minneapolis: Augsburg, 1990), 114–117; Joel Marcus, *Mark 1-8: A New Translation with Introduction and Commentary* (Garden City: Doubleday, 2000), 354–373.

I should note at the outset that this is not given to us primarily as a theological account of medicine. As is true of the gospels as a whole and the particular units of narrative or instruction in them, their primary purpose is to prompt and then answer the question: who is this man? What is this authority that he has, from where does it come, and what is its significance? And in that regard, the fact that this healing story is 'sandwiched' between the beginning and the end of a story of Jesus' raising a girl from the dead is instructive (Mk. 5:21-24, 35-43). For this complex unit is the story of *two* resurrections: one from physical death, the other from that death-in-life that an intractable illness such as this woman's comprises. That last point only makes sense in the context of the religious and social life of Israel and the way it is shaped by the instructions of Leviticus (more on that in a moment). The unit as a whole, then, is intended to leave us standing with the first witnesses of these events, amazed at Jesus' life-giving power over death. But it also serves to show us the quality of that life that Jesus came to bring: a life of *shalom*, in which people are restored to bodily integrity, life in community and relationship with God. While we need to recognize that medicine does not serve as a contemporary version of the healings of Jesus (let alone a replacement for them), this story does, nonetheless, help us see something of the nature of the plight of human vulnerability and of the healing and restoration that God intends and of which Jesus' healings and our endeavours are a prolepsis and anticipation and sign (in importantly different ways). Seeing that, however, requires a grasp of the extent of the woman's plight and the radical nature of Jesus' actions which, in turn, requires an understanding of the theological and cultural context of first-century Judaism.

The woman is described as having a 'discharge (or flow) of blood' (*rhysei haimatos*), and one that was intractable to medical treatment of the day. Twelve years intractable. Now this is no trivial matter. It would have disrupted every aspect of her life: physical, social, and 'spiritual'. Doctors are familiar with the first. Long-term menorrhagia is an uncomfortable, messy, debilitating condition – especially in a relatively poor community such as the Roman province of Judea. Most people were engaged in subsistence agriculture, with a small artisan class. As such, their livelihood depended on the vagaries of crops (if they owned a plot of land) or of the agricultural labour market (if they did not). They lived a day-to-day existence, as evidenced in both the petition of the

Lord's prayer and the parable of the workers in the vineyard (Matt. 6:9–13; 20:1–16). Theirs was an economically marginal existence. For a woman – already marginalized from the system of production – to suffer periodic bleeding for *twelve years* would almost certainly mean anaemia and malnutrition. It would also, of course, be at least uncomfortable, if not painful, depending on the underlying pathology (uterine fibroids or polyps, perhaps, or an underlying – or superimposing – infection, possibly even iatrogenic if Mark's detail in v.26 is to be trusted). Chronically fatigued, economically marginalized (due, no doubt, to a reduced capacity to work, as well as the cost of expensive and useless medical treatment), her involvement in social affairs would have been seriously compromised. We don't know if she was married – although it is telling that no husband or son is mentioned in any of the accounts – she certainly could not have performed one of her key social functions in a patriarchal culture such as Judea: she would have been barren, at least for those twelve years (reproductive physiology prohibits a menstruating woman from conceiving, of course). Her illness would have clearly compromised her engagement and standing in her community. This would have only been exacerbated by her standing under the Law. For Leviticus makes plain that a menstruating woman is unclean for the period of her menstruation and that of her cleansing afterwards (Leviticus 12 and 15). She would, as a result, be restricted in her social interactions: she herself would be 'unclean' (that is, ritually excluded from normal social affairs and especially from worship); so would anyone who touched a bed or couch on which she had sat, or who had sexual intercourse with her. She was also excluded from the religious life of Israel: she could neither go to worship in the Temple nor engage in those (relatively few) religious matters that were open to a woman in first-century Judea. And the traditions that operated in Judaism at the time (especially its stricter, Pharisaic forms) further exacerbated her plight, for out of a misguided attempt to fence the Law from any possibility of disobedience, they extended the 'infectious' nature of her uncleanness to anyone or anything she touched. Given the symbolic associations of ritual impurity, hers is a life lived as death.[28]

[28] For this, see my treatment of ritual purity in Sloane, *At Home in a Strange Land*, 113–128.

Her illness alienated her from every aspect of human bodily life in community. She was physically compromised, socially isolated and stigmatized, and excluded from normal participation in religious life. Jesus' healing of her reverses all of that. First, and most immediately (almost automatically and magically), her physical ailment is healed. And she knows it immediately, as does Jesus. But it is clear from what follows that Jesus' purpose encompasses more than physical healing, and shows the way that physical well-being is a component of and contributor to a bigger picture of flourishing. For if physical healing were all that mattered, Jesus could go on his way, not pausing on an urgent mission to deal with a relatively trivial thing. After all, she is just a woman, and she just has menorrhagia, and he's on his way to heal (indeed, raise from the dead) an important man's beloved daughter. Of course, the very fact that he pauses as he does shows that those are not his values, that he does not see her as 'just' a woman, or her condition as 'just' menorrhagia. She, too, is a daughter of Israel; hers, too, is a return from death to life. But more is going on, as is evident in the fact that at the end of the incident he pronounces her, not just healed (*hygiés*), but *whole*, even *saved* (*sesóken*). We need to remember that her plight is more than physical. Her condition has alienated her from her community and from public participation in their corporate relationship with God. Jesus' seemingly humiliating action in drawing public attention to her breach of the normal rules of social engagement and ritual purity functions as a public demonstration of the reversal of her condition and so as an act that restores her to community. She is not just physically well, she has been restored to that measure of *shalom* available to a woman in Jesus' day.

What, then, does this tell us theologically about medicine? It reminds us, first, of the nature of the disruption/s caused by disease and illness. A biomedical mindset can easily fall into the trap of considering illness to be a primarily physical ailment. We need to remember the way that illness alienates people from their bodies and interferes with their capacity to engage in the ordinary business of life. Phenomenologists of illness have reminded us of this matter;[29] the gospels (and the Psalms before them) saw this very clearly. While some aspects of the particular forms of alienation endured in biblical times are

[29] See my discussion of this in Chapter 4.

no longer relevant to us and our concerns (ritual purity is not an issue in Western culture – although we should, perhaps, remember its importance in other contemporary cultural contexts). That, in turn, reminds us that when we are engaged in medical practice, one of our goals is to restore people's ability to engage in meaningful life and relationships – to flourish – and so remove those impediments to that functioning that we reasonably can. But the nature of Jesus' action also reminds us of the importance of care and of human dignity. Medicine, even modern medicine with all its technical efficacy, can at times be an instrument of alienation rather than restoration; it can cost people much in time and money and pain and inconvenience, and leave them worse off than they were before – even if they are 'physically better'.[30] But we also need to remember that this is a story about *Jesus*, and his demonstration of the Kingdom of God and of God's final purposes for us and creation. We are not Jesus; our actions are generally not the powerful unmasking of the eschatological rule of God. Ours are efforts we make to live and work in anticipation of the final fulfilment of God's purposes for the world, done in God's name, and seeking to see God's power and compassion at work. And so any restoration to health or well-being we effect is going to be partial and provisional and temporary at best. And often, we will be 'defeated' by illness; and our patients will eventually die as, indeed, will we. In the face of that reality, we need to imitate the character of Jesus, caring for people in their vulnerability, seeking to show them and others the dignity that inheres in them as a human creature, whatever their weakness and frailty, and act in compassion whatever the outcome. In so doing, we will include the sick and weak and vulnerable in our common communal life rather than abandoning them to illness and isolation and death.

30 And, of course, if we need it, Atul Gawande, *Being Mortal: Medicine and What Matters in the End* (New York: Metropolitan Books, 2014) reminds us that much of what is done to 'care' for the elderly and dying is particularly prone to providing 'services' that do little to benefit them and their life goals and often leaves them worse off than they were before.

8

Human Vulnerability and the Goods of Medicine

Having discussed the state of medicine, philosophical and theological responses to it, and established a conceptual framework in which to understand it, it is time, at last, to directly address the questions at the heart of this project: 'What is medicine?' and 'What is it for?' I will do this by considering medicine as a social practice, locating it in the context of a Christian understanding of humanity and human community. This will necessitate figuring out what medicine is about, what goals lie at the heart of this enterprise and justify the expenditure of time, energy, resources and skill required to keep it going (the 'internal goods' towards which this social practice is oriented). As hinted at or mentioned a few times already, this will involve the counter-intuitive proposal that medicine is not, in the end, about health; it is, rather, a way in which responsible human communities care for their members as vulnerable, embodied, mortal creatures. This, in turn, will lead to an examination of the moral goods entailed in the practice of medicine, the 'internal' or inherent morality of this social practice which, while reflecting broader ethical norms, evidences its own uniqueness as a *profession*, and demonstrates that ethical issues and related theological concerns (including those related to the doctor's conscience) are not illegitimate imports into or impositions on a value-neutral expression of technical expertise, but are constitutive of medicine as a caring enterprise. While these organizing motifs will not allow me to exhaustively explore a theology of medicine, they will, I believe, enable me to present a coherent and reasonably comprehensive account of the nature and ends of medicine, one that will prove fruitful in exploring some of the moral and institutional questions that medicine needs to face.

Medicine as social practice

There is nothing new in understanding medicine as a social practice. The concept has been used in theology and philosophy of medicine since its popularization in the work of Alasdair MacIntyre, largely because of the way it illuminates medicine as an inherently moral practice and the virtues that attend its exemplary practice. As a result, much of this discussion focuses on questions of medical ethics, especially the role of the virtues in medicine as a professional practice, rather than directly and specifically addressing questions of the nature and goals of the enterprise. I will attend to questions of the inherently moral character of medicine shortly, but my focus here is on what light MacIntyre's work can shed on an understanding of medicine itself. I will begin with a brief exploration of the nature of social practices, the traditions that they bear and which nurture them, before I turn to how that helps us understand medicine as a social enterprise.

MacIntyre's widely quoted description of a social practice is worth reproducing here:

> By a 'practice' I am going to mean any coherent and complex form of socially established cooperative human activity through which goods internal to that form of activity are realized in the course of trying to achieve those standards of excellence which are appropriate to, and partially definitive of, that form of activity, with the result that human powers to achieve excellence, and human conceptions of the ends and goods involved, are systematically extended.[1]

This description or definition of a social practice was developed in the context of his discussion of late modern ethics and the loss of the traditions that inform moral reasoning and allow for or inhibit communication about ethical matters in public discourse.[2] It has, however, been used in a number of different contexts to inform our thinking about health care, especially medicine and

[1] Alasdair MacIntyre, *After Virtue: A Study in Moral Theory*, 2nd edn. (Notre Dame: University of Notre Dame Press, 1984), 187.

[2] For further, stringent criticisms of the state of public ethics and an analysis of what MacIntyre sees as intractable disagreements about questions of justice, see *Whose Justice? Which Rationality?* (London: Duckworth, 1987).

nursing.[3] While his notion of a social practice and its role in ethical reasoning has been subjected to critique and development, including whether it fosters epistemological relativism or allows for meaningful dialogue across the lines of tradition, much of that discussion has focused on its significance for our understanding of ethics *per se* and associated epistemological questions, and so has little bearing on the discussion at hand.[4] The key notions for our purpose are: a social practice as a 'coherent and complex form of socially established cooperative human activity'; 'ends and goods' and their evolution in relation to particular practices; and standards of excellence being connected with the pursuit of those ends.

Medicine is fairly clearly a highly complex form of social activity which has complex 'internal' and 'external' relationships; many of those external relationships overlap with a number of related disciplines. This raises the question of whether this complex set of institutions and social arrangements can be distinguished from related disciplines in such a way that it constitutes a social practice. I mentioned earlier the difficulty (I would say impossibility) of clearly demarcating medicine from such things as nursing, psychology, and so on, and the anxieties this might generate as to whether medicine counts as a discipline in its own right. This anxiety can be alleviated, paradoxically, by the recognition that few, if any, disciplines have the clear boundaries that the Enlightenment taught us to expect from 'sciences', and that there is no set of criteria the presence of which counts as necessary and sufficient proof that such and such a phenomenon counts as an example of such and such a discipline.

The requirement that disciplines need clear lines of demarcation or definitive criteria cannot be satisfied, and so cannot in turn be used as a criterion to determine whether something counts as a 'discipline'. Consequently, the fuzziness of the boundaries between medicine and related practices cannot be used to undermine the notion of medicine as a social practice. Disciplines are identified not by definition or demarcation but by paradigms or exemplars.

3 See, for instance, Allen Verhey, The Doctor's Oath – and a Christian Swearing It, in *On Moral Medicine: Theological Perspectives in Medical Ethics*, ed. M. Therese Lysaught et al. (Grand Rapids: Eerdmans, 2012); Mary Molewyk Doornbos, Ruth E. Groenhout, and Kendra G. Hotz, *Transforming Care: A Christian Vision of Nursing Practice* (Grand Rapids: Eerdmans, 2005), esp. 40–66.

4 For a brief discussion of some of these issues, see Andrew Sloane, *On Being a Christian in the Academy: Nicholas Wolterstorff and the Practice of Christian Scholarship* (Carlisle: Paternoster, 2003), 170–172.

Examining the behaviour of objects in motion or of fundamental particles are exemplars of the practice of physics, just as examining the behaviour of animals or of intracellular processes are exemplars of biology. But even in the 'basic' sciences, there are no clear cut boundaries between the disciplines. Molecular biology is a case in point: as the very name suggests, it necessarily involves investigation and understanding of the overlapping territories of biology, evolutionary theory, physics, physical chemistry, and so on.[5] Even so, there are clear examples of physics and biology (and so on) which help us figure out what physics and biology *are*, even if they don't allow us to police the borders between them. Medicine has such exemplary or paradigmatic practices which help us to figure out the kind of discipline it is; as Pellegrino and Svenaeus have shown, these focus on the clinical encounter exemplified in a patient's visiting their GP.[6]

These paradigmatic instances of the practice of medicine give us a sense of its unity as a social practice; they also demonstrate its complexity. Let's consider a relatively straightforward GP visit. A young woman in Australia makes an appointment to see her GP complaining of pain in her right knee, worse when walking. Having made the appointment, she tells the doctor the story of her complaint, and the doctor examines her leg. Nothing obvious appears on physical examination, except, perhaps, that her patella seems looser than normal, so she orders a set of X-rays to exclude obvious bone or joint damage. The X-rays are reported as normal, except for evidence of a hyper-mobile patella. The doctor prescribes a mild anti-inflammatory for use when needed and refers her to a physiotherapist for a short course of treatment. He examines her, manipulates her knee and prescribes a course of exercises and the use of orthotics which, over the course of a month, resolves the issue. This is a fairly uncomplicated consultation with a happy ending. But a little reflection shows that even this is a complex matter.

Leaving aside the sophisticated infrastructure that allows for easy communication and transport (say, phone calls to make appointments,

5 This is both more than and other than the fairly banal observation that higher-level and more complex phenomena (such as biological systems) incorporate the simpler and more basic phenomena that physics, say, investigates. Rather, molecular biology specifically integrates the different domains of physics, chemistry, biology, and so on. See G. Phleiderer, G. Brahier, and K. Lindpaintner (eds.), *GenEthics and Religion* (Basel: Krager, 2010).

6 See my discussions of their work in Chapters 4 and 5.

referrals and so on; buses or trains or cars for relatively rapid transport of someone not able to walk great distances, with all the advanced technology involved), this is a complex social and technological phenomenon. The patient must be aware of an institutional framework that allows her to have relatively easy (and affordable) access to a trusted professional. She needs to also have at least tacit understanding of the existence of standards of knowledge and skill that enable her to trust her GP to treat her appropriately. There have to *be* such standards and systems to ensure a reasonable level of knowledge and skill is attained before someone can set up their practice; and these must both be present and *be seen* to be present in order for there to be the level of trust required for a person in need to bring their need to another for help. There must be then, a system of training and registration, along with the complex educational (and technical) arrangements that allow for the transfer (and growth) of medical knowledge. Furthermore, at the practice level there needs to be a staff of secretaries and others that enables the practice to run. At the local level sophisticated diagnostic facilities also need to be available – generally requiring knowledge and skill both beyond and other than that of a GP – that enable X-rays, blood tests, and so on, to be performed and some guidance as to their interpretation to be given to the GP.[7] Professional alliances need to be in place so that a GP knows (or can find out) who might be the person best suited to meet more specialized needs of their patient, and systems in place that allow the patient to access those services, be they specialist medical, psychiatric or surgical services, or 'allied' health-care services such as physiotherapy, occupational therapy, psychologists and so on. These systems include funding arrangements that allow for a person with restricted income to access these facilities (a matter which is, if course, laden with political freight, especially in the US and, increasingly, the UK and Australia). And I could go on. Medicine, it is safe to say, is a complex form of cooperative social interactions involving multiple 'internal' and 'external' professional relationships that aims at particular outcomes.

[7] This was forcefully brought to my attention during a brief student placement in a hospital in north India. While it had some X-ray, haematology and biochemistry resources, they were basic and many required the doctors themselves to run them. As we are all aware, medicine is practised in many contexts where access to even those limited diagnostic facilities is unavailable.

It also has standards of excellence which it develops, monitors, evaluates and passes on to subsequent generations of practitioners, as is typical of professions, the presence, and public knowledge of and trust in which are necessary for its proper function. Both the notion of 'profession' and its application to medicine have been both criticized and defended, in part due to the ways in which it is associated with social control (of members of the 'guild' and who can/not become a member and on what terms, and of society more generally).[8] I will return to some of the questions associated with medicine as profession in relation to consumerist approaches to health care and the notion of an inherent ethics of medicine. What is relevant at this stage of the discussion is not what a 'profession' *is* and how a profession is to be distinguished from other socially valuable jobs, but whether medicine is a profession in ways that, say, being a bureaucrat is not, and in what ways might that matter. The point at issue is the notion of a social practice and the ways in which such practices govern the behaviour of both practitioners and beneficiaries of those practices. While a case can, no doubt, be made for things ranging from bureaucracy to plumbing to be understood as social practices, medicine seems not only to differ from them in crucial ways, but does so in ways that are morally and philosophically significant. The key issues here are the kinds of need that bring a patient to a doctor, the kind of power differential that exists between doctor and patient, and the kind of trust this evokes from the patient and the trustworthiness that is thereby incumbent on the doctor. The needs that turn a person into a patient strike more or less directly at their capacities to function as an embodied person in community and require the application of specialist knowledge and skill to enable them to return, if possible, to a reasonable level of functioning (more on this shortly). And the knowledge and skill required both to understand and to care for these needs, and the wisdom and even character to know how best to do so, demand standards of excellence for which we hold medical practitioners to account. The excellences of medicine must include knowledge and wisdom, technical skill and care, even love for people: these are excellences that entail more than (but not other than) a concern for technique.

[8] For useful reflections on the nature of 'professions', see Sarah Banks and Ann Gallagher, *Ethics in Professional Life: Virtues for Health and Social Care* (Basingstoke: Palgrave Macmillan, 2009), esp. 13–16, 20–23, 46–48.

Obviously there are a number of important questions that we could pursue in thinking of medicine as a social practice, to some of which I will return. However, my focus for now is on the question of the ends of medicine, as that is crucial to understanding what medicine *is*, and so what it might look like to be an exemplary practitioner of it, and how that might in turn inform our understanding of its inherent morality. This is an important set of questions, for much of the confusion and wrong-thinking about medicine is a result of either a failure to consider the internal goods of medicine or a wrong view of what those goods are. But it is equally important to recognize that answers to these questions are contextual and normative, rather than timeless or merely descriptive.

A social practice account of medicine recognizes that modern medicine, like all other human intellectual endeavours and cultural projects, is time-bound and context-dependent. Such an approach clearly differs from those like Pellegrino (and, differently, Cameron), who believe that there is a single, fixed, almost non-contingent notion of medicine and its ends.[9] As Wolterstorff notes, social practices vary across time and communities, such that their goals or ends are situation-specific.[10] Consider medicine: seventeenth-century Western medicine prescribed cupping for a number of ailments caused by an imbalance of humours. Medical excellence involved knowing the supporting theory, identifying the conditions in which it was required, and performing phlebotomy efficiently. Or, less risibly, twenty years ago the treatment of choice for gastric ulcer was medication to reduce gastric acidity and surgery, where required (say, partial gastrectomy and vagotomy). It is now directed to identifying *Helicobacter pylori* and, when present, treating it with antibiotics. We need not, however, be unduly concerned by this. First, because all knowledge and action based upon it is contingent and contextual. We can only be faulted for failures in the governing of our doxastic practices, not for having false beliefs.[11] Phlebotomized patients were harmed (in as much as their physicians' actions made them worse not better), but they were not wronged (in as much as this harm was the result of neither malice nor culpable negligence).[12] Thus the ends of social practices

9 Again, see Chapter 5 above.
10 Sloane, *On Being a Christian in the Academy*, 170–172.
11 See my discussion in Chapter 7.
12 For a helpful discussion of this distinction and its significance, see Nicholas Wolterstorff, *Justice: Rights and Wrongs* (Princeton: Princeton University Press, 2008); *Justice in Love* (Grand Rapids: Eerdmans, 2011).

such as medicine, and excellences associated with them, are contingent and contextual, at least in as much as understandings of the world and how we are to live in it influence our understanding of the proper ends of our activities and how we should attain them. Second, and more important, however, there is an overarching end that governs the small and local and larger and more general ends of medicine and which transcends in important ways the historical particularities of forms of medical practice. This can be seen in the rationale for phlebotomy, gastric surgery and antibiotics: they were conducted on the basis of available knowledge with the aim of benefiting patients.

So too, it inevitably involves normative judgements that are, in turn, driven by a broader life-and-world view. There can be no 'free-standing' evaluation of the nature and goals of medicine, for the nature and justification of medicine as a practice depends upon an underlying understanding of humanity and the goods proper to our existence as humans.[13] So, this understanding of medicine as a social practice does not emerge 'naturally' from reflection on the practice of medicine or the experience of illness and medical care or the nature of the clinical encounter; rather, it emerges from a theological account of the nature of human existence and of our calling to live in God's world, and our location of medicine in that theological context.[14] The phenomenological analysis is consistent with that perspective and helps us understand the actual practice of medicine to an extent; but the theological framework elucidates and justifies it as a practice and helps us understand the goods internal to it.

Thus, a social practice analysis can help us see the goods internal to a practice such as medicine, in such a way as to identify the implicit or explicit goods that govern it. As a number of critics have pointed out, medicine as a social practice now seems to be governed by 'goods' of technical mastery such that the use of scientific and social power for control (be that autonomy or the state) is seen to be the proper goal of medicine. This is deeply problematic from a Christian point of view. Clearly, as we have seen, that critique, and the alternative set of goods and goals I propose, emerge not from a 'neutral' observation of the phenomena of medicine, but from a normative

13 As Neil Messer has helpfully explored, for which see Chapter 6 above.

14 This, then, significantly modifies Pellegrino and Thomasma's theory in which Christian reflections on medicine are appended to a prior philosophical account (see Chapter 5).

understanding of medicine as it is located as a particular expression of key elements of how humans ought to operate in communities so as to ensure the flourishing of its members (and, for that matter, of other communities more or less distant to us in space and [future] time). While medical practitioners and policy makers need to consider how their decisions affect the lives of those 'covered' by their systems, they are part of a complex social and political system which is deeply connected with other societies in a 'global economy' and with future communities who inherit the social and economic arrangements and environmental conditions we leave them.

Hence, an understanding of the nature and ends of medicine as a social practice requires that we locate that understanding in the context of an overarching view of human life in community and what counts as flourishing in relationship. As we have seen, a biblical-theological framework allows us to see medicine as an expression of a community's care for its members whose inherent frailty and vulnerability is exposed by biological or psychological phenomena (insults to their physical or psychological health, we might say) that interfere with their ability to function meaningfully in relationships. Let me try to put that systematically.

Medicine *is* an expression of a community's commitment to care for those whose weakness as embodied creatures has been exposed by physical or psychological ailments (be they due to disease, trauma, or abnormality) and whose ability to function in meaningful relationships is thereby compromised. Its *goal* is to care for vulnerable people in such a way as to enable them to function as members of their community as well as can be reasonably expected. It is one form that a community's commitment to caring in solidarity for the weak takes, rather than abandoning them to their fate. It is a social practice that brings specialized knowledge and skill to bear on caring for vulnerable people. Its current shape is a product of modern scientific knowledge, technological skill and is shaped and misshaped by them and the bureaucratic and economic forces at work in late modern capitalism, and so it needs to be reshaped so as to better express its fundamental nature and goal, and so return caring relationship to its rightful place at the centre of the practice. At its heart is the caring relationship between doctor and patient in which the weakness of the patient is met by the power of the doctor's knowledge and skill. Such care may take the form of application of knowledge and skill and appropriate resources aimed at overcoming these limitations or healing the ailment. It may also take the form of enabling them to cope with the limitations on their relational functioning imposed by their ailment so as to maximize their ability to engage in meaningful relationships in community. It will frequently take the form of educating patients about their condition or ways of reasonably avoiding disease. While this is often driven by economic concerns, properly understood it is a way of caring for vulnerable embodied people so as to avoid unnecessary interference with their ability to function well in community. Of course, this has advantages for the community, as it reduces disease burden and enhances their communal resources. But it is still best understood as a form of care. Appropriate medical care also requires the recognition of the limits of human finitude and the corresponding inability to 'cure' those who are permanently disabled or those who are dying. This entails refraining from medicalizing both disability and the process of dying, but rather caring for people with disability so as to enable them to function in relationships as well as can be reasonably expected, and for the dying to be cared for in such a way that they can live in relationship as well as possible while they are dying. There are many areas of overlap between medicine and other aspects of a community's commitment to caring for its members, such as ancillary health care, social work, psychology, social policy and social services in general. Nonetheless, medicine has particular concerns that delineate it as a social practice even if there are no clear lines of demarcation.

Medicine as caring for this frail flesh: human vulnerability and the practice of medicine

This account differs in significant ways from how the goals and nature of medicine are normally understood. It seems obvious that 'health' is the goal of medicine, what medicine is *for*. Medicine is a crucial component of health care; it is a (paradigm) healing profession; patients go to the doctor when they feel ill, or are concerned about their health and they aim to leave well, on the road to recovery, or with their fears alleviated; we want to spend our health-care dollars to good effect, which we normally think of as being an improvement in people's health and well-being and that of our communities; most discussions of bioethics and medicine start with or at least include a discussion of health and/or healing. I could go on, but I think the point has been made.

While this seems both obvious and plausible on the face of it, it won't work for reasons I've noted a few times already. Health is not the kind of concept that can bear this degree of disciplinary weight. If it's a *concept* at all, it is a 'fuzzy' concept with imprecise boundaries and uncertain content. This makes it hard for it to function as the defining feature and overarching goal for a practice as complex and important as medicine. Furthermore, using it as a way of measuring the effectiveness of treatments or policies generates confusion and risks distortion of the practices it is meant to guide. More significantly, too much of what is important in particular kinds of medicine and the general practice of medicine at particular stages of a person's life or for particular people can't be captured by the quest for health. Even more tellingly, too much of what contributes to the health and well-being of people and communities isn't the job of medicine.[15] Failing to see this risks both 'medicalizing' human experience and illegitimately subjecting areas of life to the 'disciplinary gaze' of medicine, and abandoning weak and vulnerable people to their fate when there's no prospect of healing or improving their health.[16] Attempting to see the alleviation of suffering as the point of medicine similarly fails. None of the important dimensions of health education and prevention straightforwardly relate to the alleviation of suffering; avoidance, perhaps (but even then, it's not always clear that the result of, say, a strict weight-loss regimen leads to a net decrease in suffering, certainly not if it's measured hedonically).[17] And, of course, insurmountable problems are raised in end-of-life care and the care of disabled people: for when there is no prospect of alleviating their suffering

15 Fran Baum, *The New Public Health*, 3rd edn. (South Melbourne: Oxford University Press, 2008), esp. 227–245.

16 This is especially the case at the end of life, most tellingly (and ironically) seen in the attempt to include psychological and spiritual dimensions in the descriptors of health, such that measurable outcomes can be attained and even the process of dying subjected to bureaucratic control, for which see Jeffrey P. Bishop, Biopsychosociospiritual Medicine and Other Political Schemes, *Christian Bioethics: Non-Ecumenical Studies in Medical Morality* 15, no. 3 (2009); *The Anticipatory Corpse: Medicine, Power and the Care of the Dying* (Notre Dame, IN: UNDP, 2011), 253–284.

17 I am (perhaps reprehensibly) reminded of a Seventh Day Adventist colleague who, having somewhat gleefully cited a recent Scandinavian study that showed that non-smoking, teetotal vegans (i.e., those who for whatever reason adhered to a strict Adventist health and diet programme) lived in the order of a decade longer than their peers, then added the kicker: 'Just goes to show you how long it takes to die of boredom.'

(at least to their, or onlookers' satisfaction), the risk is that they will be abandoned by the system or abandoned to an 'easy' death.

So neither health and healing nor alleviation of suffering will do. However, for medicine to be a practice, it needs ends and goals intrinsic to it. But perhaps more important than this philosophical point, it seems clear that medicine does have a point, that it does have purposes that warrant its existence, despite the more extreme criticisms of some in the public health sector. So, what 'end' helps us understand what medicine is at its best; what helps us to see what it is and ought to be in a Christian view of the world? It seems to me that precisely a Christian understanding of human existence gives us the categories we need. For we recognize ourselves as being creatures, and creatures of a particular kind: mortal and frail; embodied and imperilled; rebellious and called; facing a past of failure and sin and a future of redemption and transformation; bound in networks of relationships which, while equally flawed and even damaging, nonetheless are meant to sustain and support us. We are, in short, frail flesh, called to inhabit communities in which we express that care for each other that exemplify the character of God and his kingdom. One form that this care takes, a characteristic form in (post) modern communities, is medicine. It is an expression of our communities' care for their vulnerable members, and a demonstration of solidarity with them rather than abandoning them to the inevitable limitations and vulnerabilities of our condition. Let me spell out what I think that means for medicine and why illness, physical and mental incapacity, and so on, matter and *should* matter so much to us.

So what, then, is medicine? What is it *for*? At its heart, medicine is about caring for this frail flesh. It is a matter of engaging with needy people whose inherent vulnerability, dependence and finitude has been exposed by the exigencies of life in this world and the way it impacts us as embodied persons.[18] Hence, it deals with a person's physical and psychological conditions (such as illness, injury, infirmity and disability), whether congenital or acquired, that interfere with their capacity to navigate the world and conduct themselves in

[18] For a similar perspective to mine on health and limitations, but which focuses on the clash between autonomous individualism and a Christian recognition of limits, including age, see Dennis Sansom, Why Do We Want to Be Healthy? Medicine, Autonomous Individualism, and the Community of Faith, *Christian Scholar's Review* 23 (1994).

meaningful social and interpersonal relationships. Its aim is not to 'heal' those conditions (for some of them are not amenable to healing), nor is it to alleviate suffering (for some of them entail no suffering *per se* – that is not the form in which the condition interferes with human flourishing). Its aim is to care for the frailty of persons-as-bodies so as to demonstrate the solidarity of the community with those in need rather than withdrawal from them. That care may take the form of attempting to reverse or alleviate the conditions that interfere with their capacity to engage in the world and in relationships; it may not. It is, however, both an expression of human flourishing, in as much as the flourishing of persons and communities entails the exercise of relationships of love and justice and fidelity (irrespective of the utility of those relationships or the persons we relate to), and a means of enhancing the flourishing of persons and communities, for it enables us to be formed as persons and communities that exemplify the character of God's kingdom and aims to do what we can to assist needy people to so engage in relationships and the world.

Medicine is, then, an expression of our common humanity and of our concern to care for fellow frail human beings in need. It is not the only way such care could have been expressed (modern medicine is, to make an obvious, even banal point, a product of the Enlightenment and the progress of science and technology that it birthed), nor is it the only way that such care is expressed in a post-Enlightenment world (nursing, physiotherapy, social work all come to mind). It is, however, one vital form that such concern takes in the world as we know it. It expresses the recognition that as moral communities we cannot abandon people in their needs; but nor can we abandon them *to* medicine and its techniques. Medicine is not a way of shunting awkward people out of the light, committing them to institutions that hide their need and remove them from the community until such a time as they are (physically or psychologically) worthy to re-join us – or, if this is no longer possible, removing them permanently from it by euthanasia. Or at least it *should* not be. Rather, we entrust people to the care that medicine provides as an expression of our solidarity with them as frail and finite beings and in recognition that their current fate will come to us all. It is, in some (perhaps paradoxical?) sense a recognition of our common humanity and of the inevitability of our own demise.

Central to the practice of medicine is the clinical encounter, the actual engagement of person in need (patient) with person who might be able to meet that need and should certainly care for them in it (doctor). It involves the actual or potential or feared experience of vulnerability occasioned by embodied persons in this fallen world who experience illness, or injury, or incapacity, or infirmity, or disability. It may be the result of their own decisions, the actions of others or the vagaries of fate. It involves some 'health' problem, with 'health' (always in scare quotes, always used under erasure) being understood as a way of speaking (loosely) of how the contingencies and vicissitudes of life impair our physical and psychological capacity to navigate the (physical, interpersonal and social) world. This is the occasion of need that brings a person to see a doctor as a patient.

The doctor has the knowledge, skill, wisdom, and so on to care for them. This places them in a position of power and requires of them the responsible exercise of their abilities. The aim of the exercise is not the healing of the patient or the alleviation of their suffering *per se*. These may be means, but they are not the end. The end is to care for this person appropriately in these circumstances in which their (and our common human) frailty and finitude has been exposed. One aspect of this care, and a subsidiary goal, I suppose, is to do what can reasonably be done to restore the person's capacity to navigate their way in the world. This, of course, may take the form of 'healing' their condition or alleviating their suffering. That is, however, one form that medical care takes (and a crucial one); it is not the only form of such care. Furthermore, it is restricted by the limitations of human finitude. Their doctor, like all doctors, has limited knowledge, skill and medical capabilities; the community has limited resources and limited medical resources (medicine is, after all, one of a number of areas of shared communal responsibility); the patient is limited in their capacity to 'recover' and to withstand the (physical, personal, relational and financial) costs of treatment. And, of course, for all its power and glory, medicine is an inherently, necessarily, inevitably tragic discipline. Infirmity, decay and death are our common fate, this side of the *eschaton*. There are limits to what we can and should do in our attempt to 'cure' the patient's condition.

So, then, health and healing and the alleviation of suffering, important as they are, are neither the aim of medicine nor its defining feature. When the limits of cure are reached, we are not left with a different kind of medicine, let alone a different practice altogether; rather, we need to express a different form of the point of medicine: caring for this frail flesh. That care, whatever form it takes, is a demonstration of our solidarity with needy people rather than their abandonment. When 'cure' is possible (or feasible), this care-in-solidarity takes the form of 'healing' (subject to its limitations); when 'cure' is not possible it takes a different form – support, amelioration of symptoms, staring together at the approaching face of death, trusting and hoping in the fidelity of the God of resurrection. The goal is simply this: to so care for this person's frail flesh that they are enabled to function (as persons and in relationship) as well as they reasonably can in the circumstances they find themselves facing, and so to express what human community looks like on those occasions when our common frailty and finitude is exposed by the vicissitudes of embodied life in a fallen world.

The goods associated with that end are, I suppose, 'health'-related goods. To relieve suffering where suffering is a problem and impinges on human flourishing; to heal disease when that impinges on human flourishing; to care. The latter re-humanizes medicine, requiring a focus on the patient's story, the recognition of both the need for and limits of the doctor's focus on 'disease' and so on. It requires the embrace of those who would otherwise experience the alienation and disruption of illness, infirmity, trauma or the inevitable decay of their organismic capacities, rather than their abandonment. It is, interestingly, a fitting way to resist the draw of total care and the medicalization of ordinary human experience. For it recognizes the clear limitations of medical care and that some things are not in its purview; it recognizes that medicine is an important expression of the community's care for its members – but only one such expression, and so leaves room for others; it recognizes that, paradoxically, totalizing medicine is a form of abandonment, of renouncing our personal and communal responsibilities for each other, outsourcing it to the clinic or hospice or asylum (or 'thanatorium'), and so excluding those who most need our embrace.

It is important, however, to recognize that 'health' functions adjectivally rather than nominally in our understanding of medicine. That is to say, it is a descriptor of the form or quality of care medicine provides, that care being the 'whatness' of medicine. Medicine is not about *health* care, but about 'health' *care*, that is, care which focuses on vulnerabilities of human embodied existence – the care of this frail flesh. We must, then, recognize that 'health' is a 'fuzzy concept' and that it is unnecessary to define it or determine which of health, disease or illness has priority. For medicine is about 'caring for this frail flesh' and health, disease and illness are rough-and-ready ways of picking out the kinds of things we're concerned about rather than defining what they are. This is important to remember in relation to public policy and the analysis of the effectiveness of medical treatment. 'Health' is not a 'thing' or concept, or even a composite state subject to a general metric. Metrics can be used with respect to, say, cardiac function and the capacity to engage in tasks of everyday life; and some (even meaningful) comparisons can be made, say, between the incapacities generated by cardiac or pulmonary or renal failure. I don't see, however, that we can then meaningfully speak of a general 'health index' in which we compare the relative dysfunction that results from particular conditions, or the benefits of particular treatments. Such indices are conceptually confused and practically dangerous attempts to universalize particular descriptions, and (statistically) compare and measure incommensurables. This, of course, raises significant problems for the use of a QALY (or Disability Adjusted Life Year [DALY]) index in public policy or the measurement of treatment efficacy, especially as they almost inevitably disadvantage disabled people and others who are already socially disadvantaged. Perhaps something like a QALY index can be used as a rough way of figuring out the relative utility of particular treatments for particular people; nonetheless, we cannot transfer that to other population groups or even classes of patients, as the base levels are so different. Meaningful comparison requires comparing like with like; but such health metrics can only work by erasing the particularities of circumstances and patients and conditions. Policy decisions need to be made on other grounds and need to be explicit about the (kinds of) value judgements that inevitably drive them. And there the Scriptures clearly have something to say.

In passing, I wonder whether this perspective might help explain the puzzling, even ironic, effects of the focus on 'health-care efficiency' in the last five to ten years. Bureaucratic control has increased dramatically, along with the administrative and paperwork burden, without demonstrable improvement in services (indeed, often to the detriment of care, especially for the vulnerable). This may be because bureaucracies tend to have particular interests and values which, while they may be goods internal to the practice of bureaucracy, are not those goods that govern medical practice and so these interests and values do not line up with those of the systems they are meant to manage.[19] In relation to this, 'efficiency' only works if it is rightly directed. Imagine a car. Its purpose is to take us from one place to another. If we spend all our time on improving speed, fuel efficiency, and so on, but we fail to consider the direction we're going, all the improvements in efficiency may serve no purpose or even worsen our plight – taking us further and faster away from our proper goal. So, I suspect, with bureaucratically driven health care. Furthermore, some crucial elements of medicine are clearly *not* subject to utilitarian calculus, particularly those relating to end of life care.[20]

Interestingly, focusing on cutting costs/utility/efficiency, like focusing on population control, is likely to be less effective, paradoxically, than focusing on basic equity and a decent minimum of care. The latter is intrinsically right and, incidentally, best ensures good (and cost-effective) outcomes and achieves the desired end (demographic conversion in relation to population, improvements in health at the population level).[21] This, of course, adds force to arguments to allow the internal goods of medicine to control its practice rather than cost or efficiency. Mind you, for Christian theology, efficiencies and utilitarian metrics are unlikely to be driving forces. Most discussions of the economics of health-care allocation (particularly in relation to the elderly) operate using a logic alien to the gospel and antithetical to the claims of the universal lordship of Christ.[22] We need a different justification such that rationing, where and when

19 Michael Loughlin et al., Philosophy, Medicine and Health Care – Where We Have Come From and Where We Are Going, *Journal of Evaluation in Clinical Practice* 20 (2014): 902–903.

20 For this, see Bishop, Biopsychosociospiritual Medicine and Other Political Schemes; *The Anticipatory Corpse*, 253–278.

21 For this, see Baum, *The New Public Health*, 16, 227–245; Lisa Sowle Cahill, *Theological Bioethics: Participation, Justice, Change* (Washington, DC: Georgetown University Press, 2005), 131–168, in relation to health, and Susan Power Bratton, *Six Billion and More: Human Population Regulation and Christian Ethics* (Louisville: Westminster/John Knox, 1992), esp. 29–39, 138–174 on justice and education as the most effective means of population control.

22 See, for instance, Alvin H. Moss and Mark Siegler, Should Alcoholics Compete Equally for Liver Transplantation?, in *Bioethics: An Anthology*, ed. Helga Kuhse and Peter Singer (Oxford: Blackwell, 2006); Robert M. Veatch, How Age Should Matter: Justice as the Basis for Limiting Care to the Elderly, in *Bioethics: An Anthology*, ed. Helga Kuhse and Peter Singer (Oxford: Blackwell, 2006); Norman Daniels, A Lifespan Approach to Health Care, in *Bioethics: An Anthology*, ed. Helga Kuhse and Peter Singer (Oxford: Blackwell, 2006); and for the need for a Christian perspective, see Some Issues and the Future of Theological Reflection: Reports of the Working Groups, in *Religion and Medical Ethics: Looking Back, Looking Forward*, ed. Allen Verhey (Grand Rapids: Eerdmans, 1996); Joel Shuman and Brian Volck, *Reclaiming the Body: Christians and the Faithful Use of Modern Medicine* (Grand Rapids: Brazos, 2006), 94–10; D. Stephen Long, The Language of Death: Theology and Economics in Conflict, in *On Moral Medicine: Theological Perspectives in Medical Ethics*, ed. M. Therese Lysaught et al. (Grand Rapids: Eerdmans, 2012).

it is necessary, is driven by a properly theological account of medicine and its role in human community.[23]

Medicine as an inherently moral practice

Consideration of medicine as a social practice and the ends and goods internal to it brings us to a consideration of the *excellences* or virtues of medicine; for evolving understandings of such excellences and their role in pursuit of the goods of a practice are fundamental to understanding social practices and their operation, including medicine. As already noted, these virtues are primarily exercises of practical wisdom, involving particular bodies of knowledge and sets of skills and the wisdom to know which element of knowledge and what set of skills to bring to bear on a particular case of human need. The inherent power differential at work (the need of the patient; the specialized knowledge and skill of the practitioner and the limits and controls placed on the technologies and so on available to a practitioner) generate obligations for the practitioner, including moral obligations. From a Christian point of view, power is a moral phenomenon that evokes its use for the good of those without it – or at least, so it should. Furthermore, at the heart of medicine is not knowledge and skill, or the use of technique, but *care*, particularly the care of human vulnerability as it is exposed in conditions of illness, injury or incapacity. It is, once again, one key way we as communities care for this frail flesh. This, in turn, means that we need to consider excellences of care. These excellences, of course, involve knowledge and skills: how humans respond to their experiences of vulnerability; how to understand their experiences and what may lie behind them; how to demonstrate that the bringing to bear of the puzzling complexities of the medical system is an expression of solidarity with this needy person, not an abandoning of them to the machinery of 'total care'; and so on. But the excellences of care are primarily *moral*. Care entails the growth in and (in part by way of) the exercise of the virtues of care.

23 I will discuss this briefly in the next chapter in relation to allocation of health-care resources and the grounds on which such decisions should be made.

Now, I must acknowledge that the shape of medical morality is a complex and vexed issue, one with a long tradition and the large body of literature that comes with it. There are many important questions that would need to be addressed in framing a comprehensive theory of medical ethics, including the role of virtues in it and which virtues are to operate and with what importance and whether, strictly speaking, it is a morality *internal* to medicine and how it might relate to general ethics and the communities with which they are connected. These are all disputed questions which have been discussed at length in treatments of medical ethics and bioethics.[24] While these are important questions, they have received a great deal of attention and they are neither the focus of my discussion, nor are they the most important matters for the theology or philosophy of medicine. Of more significance than the form medical morality might take and the relative weight of (specific) virtues or obligations or consequences and how particular they may be to medicine, is that medicine is an inherently moral enterprise and that this arises out of both its nature as a practice of care and its location in a vision of society and human flourishing. And that is my concern. In this regard, it is vital to note that a doctor's conscientious objection to certain procedures or policies, and questions they may have relating to the *ethics* (not just efficacy) of specific treatments are not alien concerns imported into medical practice by conservative practitioners, but are fundamental to the moral agency of doctors which is, in turn, of the very essence of medicine.

Note that this is an *inherent*, but *derived* morality; it emerges from a broader theological and social vision rather than being either free-standing or the product of reflection simply on how medicine is conducted as a practice. As

24 See, for instance, Edmund D. Pellegrino and David C. Thomasma, *The Christian Virtues in Medical Practice* (Washington, DC: Georgetown University Press, 1996); Banks and Gallagher, *Ethics in Professional Life: Virtues for Health and Social Care*. Useful discussions of the internal morality of medicine can also be found in Aana Vigen, Listening to Women of Color with Breast Cancer: Theological and Ethical Insights for US Healthcare; and 'Keeping it Real' while Staying Out of the 'Loony Bin': Social Ethics for Healthcare Systems, in *On Moral Medicine: Theological Perspectives in Medical Ethics*, ed. M. Therese Lysaught et al. (Grand Rapids: Eerdmans, 2012), 168–172; and see the Introduction to the chapter on the professions in M. Therese Lysaught et al (eds.), *On Moral Medicine: Theological Perspectives in Medical Ethics*, 3rd edn. (Grand Rapids: Eerdmans, 2012), 219–222, esp. the question of internal goods and virtues on p.220. And the excellent piece by Joseph J. Kotva, Jr, The Christian Pastor's Role in Medical Ethics: In the Pew and at the Bedside, in *On Moral Medicine: Theological Perspectives in Medical Ethics*, ed. M. Therese Lysaught et al. (Grand Rapids: Eerdmans, 2012); Verhey, The Doctor's Oath.

such, it is also necessarily pluralistic, for the social and moral visions that give rise to and shape medical practice are plural. While I think the understanding of medicine I've outlined here makes best sense of what medicine is and ought to be, it is unashamedly and unapologetically a *Christian* understanding, arising out of an explicitly Christian understanding of the world. That is, however, no defect, for all theoretical activity is irreducibly plural, as are the practices associated with it. We should, then, not only allow but *expect* a plurality of theory and practice in relation to medicine. This doesn't mean we're trapped in a theological and moral monastery (let alone a ghetto); the practice of Christian medicine no more necessitates a Christian institutional framework than does the practice of Christian scholarship.[25] Sometimes such a context may be useful or necessary for particular purposes, at other times not. Just as Christian education and scholarship can be conducted faithfully in a pluralistic environment, so can medicine. This may involve struggle, compromise, faithful refusal to engage in certain activities as an expression of and witness to Christian commitment. It may mean problems with advancement, or even involvement in certain institutional contexts (for instance, the recent move by the Royal College of Obstetricians and Gynaecologists in the UK to exclude those who refuse to provide contraception or abortion services on the grounds of conscience). But so be it. Sometimes we just need the courage of our convictions (as the cliché goes), and the willingness to pay their price.

25 James Rusthoven, *Covenantal Biomedical Ethics for Contemporary Medicine: An Alternative to Principles-Based Ethics* (Eugene, OR: Pickwick, 2014) has a good discussion of these issues.

9

Re-engaging the World of Medicine: Applying Philosophy and Theology of Medicine

A summary of the argument so far

Medicine, as we have seen, is a complex social practice that bears a great deal of social and moral freight. Theological and philosophical reflection on the practice of medicine has, I believe, yielded interesting fruit. It is now time to bring this discussion together and, in turn, bring it to bear on some of the bioethical questions that are raised by the practice of medicine and the issues that face medicine as a global phenomenon. Questions arising out of the global context of medicine were raised in Chapter 2 in my discussion of the recent Ebola crisis and what it shows about the nature of contemporary medical practice. The ethics of euthanasia and organ transplantation were addressed in Chapter 3. I will return to these matters shortly, re-engaging the world of medicine in light of my theological and philosophical reflections on the nature of medicine. But before I do that, it is worth revisiting my argument and summarizing my findings.

In Chapter 4, I dealt with perspectives on philosophy of medicine, focusing on the nature of health and healing, EBM and medical reasoning, and the phenomenology of medicine. Perhaps surprisingly, I contend that health and healing do not give us an adequate account of the nature and purposes of medicine due to both conceptual issues with definitions of health and related terms such as illness and disease, and the way in which medicine deals with matters other than healing, and practices other than medicine contribute substantially to the goals of health. Philosophical discussions of health are important, and matters of health are of obvious significance to the practice of medicine; but 'health and healing' do not give us an adequate framework for understanding the nature and practice of medicine. EBM raises important questions about medicine as both a clinical practice, centring on the relationship between a doctor and their patient, and a practice of inquiry, involving institutions, cultural patterns, ways of seeing the world, and so forth, aimed at understanding the world and engaging in informed patient care. EBM can certainly contribute to both knowledge and clinical practice, but it is neither an adequate nor a required basis for it. Our understanding of medical knowing needs to be person-centred and draw on clinical experience and the wisdom of tradition, careful interpretation and personal judgement. Clinical practice needs to be informed by evidence and disciplined reflection, but we need to remember that both the knowledge that medicine generates and the care that knowledge is meant to serve are person- and situation-specific. Indeed, as the phenomenology of health and medical practice shows, medicine is a fundamentally *personal* practice, focusing on people and their needs and on the relationship between a doctor, with their skill and knowledge, and a patient, in their need and dependence. This helpfully reorients our understanding of medicine away from an obsession with technical mastery and towards a concern for persons and the way that illness disrupts their ability to function as persons in the world, and a doctor's role as someone whose skill is justified by and is aimed towards caring for needy persons.

Chapter 5 turned to recent work on theology and medicine, examining the work of Pope John Paul II, Nigel Cameron and Stanley Hauerwas. The late Pope's work illustrated serious concerns that emerge from Christian reflection on the current state of medicine and the way it reflects attitudes to the weak and vulnerable and notions of human freedom deeply at odds with traditional appropriations of the Bible's witness to God's character and purposes. His theological counter-proposal to the 'culture of death' entails the articulation of an alternative view of human persons and human community; it stops short, however, of developing a theology of medicine *per se*. Cameron shares much of John Paul II's analysis of the state of medicine, arguing that in as much as it departs from the (Christianized) Hippocratic tradition of Western medicine, it has abandoned its moral foundation and is left as a mere set of technical skills and expert knowledge to be used at the whim of consumers of this product. Cameron's analysis depends on a problematic understanding of the Hippocratic tradition and its history, and of the centrality of 'health and healing' to medical practice, and fails to integrate theological reflection on the nature and practice of medicine into his discussion of the profession and its internal morality. Nonetheless, he raises important considerations regarding medicine as an inherently moral practice and the limits this places on patient autonomy.

Hauerwas presents a more overtly theological account of medicine and, despite the problems associated with his focus on the Church as an alternative community on his theology and ethics, he raises important questions that a Christian understanding of medicine must address. He believes that medicine has embraced an idolatrous goal, the attaining of technical mastery so as to overcome the limits inherent in the human condition and the inevitability of death. It has rejected the Christian story and its resources for dealing with frailty and finitude and embraced the false stories of modernity and, in so doing, medicine has lost the capacity to be an inherently moral enterprise driven by values greater and other than those of the market. His call to return care rather than cure to the centre of the understanding and practice of medicine is both salutary and coheres well with the character of the Christian story; it is also consistent with Pellegrino and Thomasma's Christian theory of medicine. Their understanding of the inherently moral character of medicine emerges from a phenomenological account of the clinical encounter. Of crucial importance is their recognition that the nature of a patient's need and of the power differential that exists between patient and doctor means medical care cannot be understood as a tradeable commodity owned by doctors (or medical institutions) and consumed by patients. It is a moral enterprise in which care meets need for the benefit of needy persons. Their theory suffers from its being rooted in a demarcationist philosophy of science that sees it as important that medicine be clearly delineated from other disciplines, and in a theological tradition in which theological reflection is overlaid on prior independent philosophical analysis. So too, they share many theorists' idea that medicine is *about* health and healing, a view that I believe misunderstands both the nature and purpose of medicine.

The question of the nature of health and its theological significance comes to the centre of the discussion in Chapter 6's examination of the work of Neil Messer. Messer presents a helpful overview of various notions of health, disease and illness and the role they play in bioethics and theories of health care, noting both the fuzziness of the concepts and the ways that many treatments of them exemplify the modernist tendency to divorce fact from value. While there are problems with how he does so, Messer also rightly incorporates disability theory into his discussion, noting the way it both critiques and enriches prevailing theories of bioethics and health care. At the heart of his discussion is a theological account of flourishing, which he sees as both distinct from health and related to it. His theological framework draws widely from the Christian tradition, paying particular attention to the work of Karl Barth and Thomas Aquinas. Messer affirms Barth's fluid notion of health as 'strength for human life', and the influence of society and political and economic systems on well-being, as well as the importance of recognizing that suffering, limitation and even death are fundamental to the human condition and must be accounted for in any theory of health (hence the role that theologies of disability play in Messer's work). He also embraces Aquinas' view that an understanding of transcendent *teloi* is necessary for a proper understanding of human creaturely existence and so of flourishing and health. Messer constructs and applies a theology of health in which bodily integrity, while a good of human life and a contributor to its flourishing, is neither the ultimate good of our existence nor *necessary* for it: human beings can find forms of flourishing in the face of disability, infirmity and even when facing death. For all the richness and fertility of Messer's theology of flourishing, I think he is mistaken to see 'health' as the key to our understanding of medicine, which prompted me to develop my own theological understanding of medicine.

In Chapter 7, I outline the philosophical and theological framework within which I believe a Christian theory of medicine can be articulated and justified. I begin with a critique of modernist theories of rationality that have dominated approaches to science, including medicine, and an outline of an alternative (non-relativist) person- and situation-specific epistemology. Integral to that epistemology is the recognition that our beliefs are, in general, innocent-until-proven-guilty. They are the product of belief-forming mechanisms in which pre-existing concepts, ways of seeing the world, and so on, give us access to the world, as well as occasionally interfering with proper knowledge of it. When we come to see that something in our cloak of beliefs and patterns of belief-formation has gone wrong we are obliged to seek to correct it and the beliefs it generated. And the more important such beliefs and mechanisms are to the projects we are called to the more important it is to carefully govern our practices of inquiry so as to increase their likelihood of being correctly aligned with the way the world is. However, the result will not be a value-neutral body of knowledge, for the beliefs and practices that shape our engagement with the world also shape what we come to believe about it and the theories we devise in order to understand it. This, contrary to modernist prejudices against particularity, is not a flaw in our theoretical endeavours, but an inevitable feature of the way finite, embodied (and, yes, sinful) beings such as we are come to know the world and reflect upon it. But it does mean that significant differences in those core (or control) beliefs will give rise to significantly different theories. For a Christian, the beliefs that are entailed in their authentic Christian commitment will and ought to play a crucial role in the shaping of their ways of understanding the world, and so, the theories they devise and accept – including theories of medicine.

The beliefs central to Christian commitment are, I believe, best understood in light of a narratively driven biblical theology. I outline such a theology and note its implications both for Christian epistemology and for a theology of medicine. Creation grounds our quest for knowledge in the orderly character of God and the world and establishes limits on the kind of technical mastery we should seek: we are finite creatures and always will be; there is no faithful escape from the exigencies of creatureliness. The brokenness of the world as it now is limits our capacity to know truly, for we are as broken as the world we seek to understand. Yet it necessitates our attempt to understand the world and shapes our efforts to change it; for the God who both made and judges the world also seeks to redeem and transform us and calls human creatures to be agents of God's work of fixing a broken world. In Jesus, we see both the clearest expression of that transforming work and the anticipation of its final state. In him, we also hear the call to be ourselves transformed and mobilized in God's great free-making mission as we work to see glimpses of our final destiny and his perfect future in our fleeting and flawed projects. Such a theological perspective requires that we understand the limits of our endeavours: any change we make to the world or needy people in it will be partial and temporary at best; we are still subject to death and the world will only be made new by the sovereign work of God, not the labour of our hands. We build signposts to that final transformation, and occasionally plant oases on the road towards it; the garden-city for which we long, and to which we seek to witness by word and deed, will be the gift of God, as is evident in the story of Jesus' healing of the woman with menorrhagia in Mark 5.

In Chapter 8, I outline my theory of medicine, drawing on notions of medicine as a social practice, and the internal goods associated with that practice, and articulating medicine as an embodiment of the care a community owes its members whose vulnerability has been exposed by way of physical or psychological malady. As a social practice, medicine has a set of institutional frameworks that foster the qualities and behaviours that count as good medical practice, train practitioners in their use and induct them into the practice, and seek to monitor and maintain standards. But those institutions and standards aim at the attaining of the goods that are internal to medicine as a profession, and which arise out of the *teloi* of this social practice. Despite the popularity of the idea that medicine's goal is health and healing and/or the alleviation of suffering, I argue that this understanding will not do. Medicine's goal is to care for vulnerable people in such a way that a doctor's personal and technical expertise is brought to bear on the patient's need (a need, in turn, which is the result of a disruption of their physical or psychological functioning) so as to restore them to a reasonable level of functioning in relationships, or to enable them to cope as well as they can with their ailment. Medicine's *goal* is to express appropriate care for vulnerable people in circumstances such as this. Medicine's *nature* is to be an expression of a community's solidarity with and care for its members whose inherent frailty has been exposed by physical or psychological disruption. Medicine *is*, so to speak, what it *does*. Or at least, that's how it should be. Of course, such an understanding of medicine is rooted in and arises out of a broader philosophical and theological vision. This is as it should be. It also requires that medicine be seen as an inherently moral enterprise. In as much as it entails the use of power for the benefit of those in need and requires a particular understanding of human flourishing that it seeks to foster, moral questions operate internally to the practice of medicine, rather than being an imposition from external religious or moral systems. While a controversial view in contemporary medical politics, I fail to see how any other understanding of medicine makes sense of the nature of medicine or the theological context that gives it its meaning.

If this understanding of the nature and purpose of medicine is right, then questions immediately arise about what kind of medical care is appropriate in what circumstances, and what justifies those decisions. These questions are of obvious relevance to the issues I raised at the start of the book: resource limitations in majority world contexts, and commodification and ballooning expectations in the West; euthanasia and end of life care, and the ethics of transplants and their relationship to what we expect – and can *rightly* expect – of medicine. So, before I return to the issues I used as doorways into the philosophy of medicine, I will outline how I believe medical care can be justified and what that implies for decisions we might make about what care is or is not appropriate.

Bringing philosophy and theology of medicine to bear on the world of practice

The nature of medicine and the ends to which it should be put

It is important at this stage to remember that our understanding of medicine and its justification is derived from a broader vision of human life in community and the nature of embodied existence. Illness is a problem because it adversely affects people and interferes with their ability to function in relationships. The justification of medicine, then, lies in its ability to do something about those factors related to disease processes, injury, or physical or psycho-social disruption which interfere with a person's ability to function in relationships, their *flourishing*. The goal of medicine has a similar relational orientation: its goal is not to 'fight disease', or to improve the health of the community: that is to mistake the *means* for the *end*. The goal of health care is to care for vulnerable people and enable them to be restored to proper functioning in their relationships and as persons, as far as this is practicable.

Not only is our understanding of medicine derived from a broader understanding of community, medicine itself exists in and for a given community as an expression of that community's care for its vulnerable members. Every society has the obligation, arising out of the implicit agreement of those who comprise it, to provide those things its members need for (at least minimal) community involvement. So, we have seen that medicine has a clear individual focus, in as much as the very essence of the clinical relationship is a person in need going to another person. But it is also corporate, because the existence of medical institutions, and the ability of medical professionals to engage in such a clinical relationship, arises out of, and is funded by, a community's commitment to meet the health needs of its members. Now, the range of health-care options available in contemporary Western societies is almost unlimited; the resources to meet the needs of people within those communities are not. Consequently, we need to figure out what kinds of services a person can rightly expect to receive, and the community rightly be expected to provide to all its members, and what services, if any, go beyond those expectations, those *entitlements*.

This notion of *entitlement* needs a little unpacking. An entitlement is, as I've already implied, something we can rightly expect to receive or have available to us, such that being deprived of it by other individuals, or by social systems and structures, counts as an infringement on our rights. To be denied what we are entitled to is to be wronged, to be treated unjustly.[1] When we then think of how human communities ought to function (be that as societies, economies or polities) and do so in light of a Christian understanding of God's desire that humans and their communities flourish, that they enjoy *shalom*, that notion of entitlement comes to bear. For a properly functioning community will ensure that its members have access to those goods and services that they need in order to engage meaningfully in community life and flourish as persons. The minimum required is what enables us to function as persons and in relationships *at all*, what we need to sustain our individual and social life. These can be called sustenance rights, such as food, water, housing, education, basic health care, and so on.[2] These are rights, because they are necessary for functioning in community; without them, people are unable to function meaningfully in relationships and pursue the ends for which they were created. Beyond these sustenance rights which societies are obliged to meet, society may choose to offer us other services, which go beyond meeting those basic

1 See Nicholas Wolterstorff, *Justice: Rights and Wrongs* (Princeton: Princeton University Press, 2008); *Justice in Love* (Grand Rapids: Eerdmans, 2011).

2 For a discussion and justification of this notion of *sustenance rights*, see Nicholas Wolterstorff, *Until Justice and Peace Embrace* (Grand Rapids: Eerdmans, 1983), 73–98. His discussion is conducted in relation to issues of international justice in the global economy but is applicable, I believe, to the provision of medical services in both the Western and the majority world.

needs. This distinction between entitlements and other services provides us with a way of determining whether and what kind of care is justified in a particular instance, especially when coupled with the recognition that the primary task of medicine is to care for people in their vulnerability.[3]

First, of course, we need to think about what kind of medical care counts as a sustenance right, an entitlement. This is a complex and situation-specific task, but remembering that medicine is an expression of a community's commitment to its vulnerable members rather than abandoning them to their fate, and that the clinical encounter between a doctor and their patient is at the heart of the practice of medicine, gives us a way forward. Broadly speaking, our sustenance health-care rights include community health resources, and the services that cluster around a good general practice, for they are a fitting expression of care for the vulnerable and are required if the relational dysfunction occasioned by illness or accident is to be overcome at all. Of course, what is included in community health care and what services are provided by a GP and the services that are integrally connected with their practice, will vary depending on historical, cultural, political and economic circumstances. It would be unreasonable for a GP in Australia in the early twenty-first century *not* to provide antibiotics to someone they suspect has pneumonia or refer them for a chest X-ray. It would be equally unreasonable to have expected a doctor in early eighteenth-century England to have done so.

Clearly, however, the range of services available in modern medicine goes well beyond the basic care offered through those services that cluster around a general practice. We need also to consider tertiary health services, the kind of care available in a teaching hospital in the West, including sophisticated diagnostic facilities, specialist surgery, intensive and coronary care, and so forth. We cannot see such care as an entitlement. ICU care, for instance, is both expensive and requires a significant level of infrastructure and personnel to support it, such that it is difficult or impossible to set up and maintain a tertiary hospital outside a major urban centre. Attempting to provide such services for

3 See Andrew Sloane, Painful Justice: An Ethical Perspective on the Allocation of Trauma Services in Australia, *The Australian and New Zealand Journal of Surgery* 68, no. 11 (1998).

rural and remote communities would beggar an economy, even an affluent one like Australia's, and would result in the loss of other essential services. Indeed, it would be self-defeating, as a tertiary hospital needs well-trained personnel, good transport services, advanced technology and communication, and so on, all of which would be compromised if we were to attempt to establish an ICU in every rural centre which would, in turn, mean that the ICU would become useless fairly quickly. Such services cannot count as basic health care; nor can they be counted as an entitlement, as attempting to provide them would interfere with the provision of (other kinds of) sustenance rights. This is not to say that they are illegitimate, that we should call an embargo on the development of sophisticated medical technologies and dismantle the facilities we already have. It just means that they are not services to which we are *entitled*. We need another category.

I'm not quite sure what to call it: something like 'health-care mercies', or 'privileges', perhaps. These are services that go beyond what members of a community are entitled to, but which a community legitimately offers its members. Tertiary hospitals are a paradigm example, it seems to me. How are we to determine what services are appropriate? Again, our understanding of medicine comes to our aid. Medicine is not about acceding to the demands and desires of people who wish to escape human finitude and mortality. Nor should it driven by 'Hippocratic beneficence', such that any treatment that might be of some benefit to this individual patient is thereby justified.[4] There are limits to what we can legitimately do, and sometimes this means that a therapy that *might* do some good for a person is withheld. And sometimes this means that they will not be cured when perhaps they could have been, and they may even die. If medicine is seen as *caring* for such people rather than providing a cure, then we have grounds both for saying that the appropriate care someone receives may not lead to their cure; and if the *therapeutic* goal of medicine is to do what we reasonably can to return someone to a reasonable level of relational functioning (when *therapy* is the appropriate form that

[4] What I have called 'Hippocratic beneficence' is (as I imply above) the notion that a doctor has the duty to provide their patient any and all treatment that is available and might do some therapeutic good. For brief discussions of this, see Painful Justice, and Christianity and the Transformation of Medicine, in *Christianity and the Disciplines: The Transformation of the University*, ed. Oliver D. Crisp et al. (London: T&T Clark, 2012), 87–88.

care should take), then we have grounds for making judgements about whether therapeutic intervention is appropriate and, if so, of which kind. If a treatment option does not offer a reasonable prospect of someone's being returned to a reasonable level of relational functioning, and if that care cannot be counted as basic care to which everyone is entitled, then it is inappropriate to provide such care. While I'm not sure that such care should be *banned* in a democratic context such as Australia (I can't see how such a law could be justly framed, and I think there's a clear difference between which uses of a person's money and resources are ethically justified and which uses should be legally permitted), it does not seem to me to be ethically warranted or theologically appropriate.

This gives us something like a set of criteria by which we can judge the theological and ethical warrant for the provision of medical services. Health-care services are justified if *either*: they are components of basic health care to which everyone is entitled as a sustenance right; *or* their provision offers reasonable hope of return to a reasonable level of relational functioning, and the provision of these services will not impinge on the provision of sustenance rights to others. This criterion allows us to always provide those basic health services which, within a given community, can be justified as sustenance rights, as well as provide just and equitable access to other resources.

Reconsidering organ transplantation

This understanding of medicine and the criteria for the provision of care has clear implications in relation to the ethics of organ transplantation. To begin with, it calls into question the way the discussion is normally framed. As we saw with Radcliffe Richards' argument, the assumption is that organ transplantation should be provided whenever possible. People with end-stage organ failure are clearly in need: their lives are severely limited by their condition and, in many cases, they face imminent death should they not receive a transplant. If medicine is about 'health and healing', then it seems obvious that life-saving organ transplantation should be provided. Re-envisioning medicine as being about caring for 'frail mortal flesh' should give us pause. It *may* be that organ transplantation is the appropriate form that care might take; but perhaps not. We must not *assume* that it is, as much contemporary discussion assumes (Radcliffe Richards is again a case in point): transplant surgery is not a health-care entitlement. It not only requires initial and ongoing access to tertiary-level medical facilities, it requires that an organ be available. Given the practical limitations of access and so on I noted earlier, and that there are fewer organs available than people who could benefit (and always will be, short of science-fiction scenarios such as cloned organs or draconian social policies), we cannot provide transplant services for everyone who might benefit.

So if organ transplantation is not an entitlement, then if it is to be justified, it must both offer a reasonable chance of a return to a reasonable level of relational functioning *and* not interfere with the provision of sustenance rights to others (be they health-care or sustenance rights). The first criterion can, I think, be satisfied for most transplant surgery in light of advances in technology and procedures. That was not the case in the early, developmental phases of transplantation (as is true for many 'experimental' therapeutic measures). The justification for such experimental therapies lies less in their being instances of medical care and more in their being instances of advances in knowledge and expertise. There are significant questions relating to the ethics of human subject research that need to be addressed, but they are quite different to the questions that need to be asked about the appropriateness of such procedures as *treatment* options. I would suggest, in passing, that our tendency to conflate these questions results in both confusion and inappropriate treatment decisions, especially when coupled with the unwarranted expectations we have and our desire to gain technical mastery over the limitations of the human condition. When Baconian technique, the unfettered human will, and the notion that medicine is about healing or the alleviation of suffering meet an emerging technology, the result can only be a sense that this needy person is entitled to this radical, exciting new treatment and is wronged if they are denied it by a heartless health-care system. Again, we need to untangle experimental medical interventions from our assumptions about appropriate medical care and think deeply about how we determine what care is appropriate. Nonetheless, it seems to me that questions of efficacy (or relational utility, if you will) can generally be satisfied in relation to transplants.

What about the question of whether provision of such services impinges on the provision of sustenance rights to others? Here, I think we need to distinguish between two questions: Should we provide such services at all? And to what extent should they be provided and to whom? Viewing transplants as a medical *mercy* (rather than a health-care entitlement) helps with both questions. For the sake of argument, I will take it as given that some provision of transplants is acceptable; and we have already seen that it cannot be made available to everyone. That means that societies, and their governments, will need to make decisions about the level of services they will provide, how they will do so, and on what terms they will be provided – including the mix of public and private medicine. My inclination is towards a mixed public and private medical system, such as we have in Australia, rather than purely a market-driven or fully socialized one, but be that as it may. The point is that such decisions must be made and, whether they include some kind of lottery or depend on a person's ability to pay, some people must miss out. And they will be harmed as a result: that is, some benefit that they would otherwise receive will be denied to them. They will not, however, be *wronged*, as none of their rights will have been infringed. It may be tragic, but such is the nature of the human condition. We are frail and mortal beings, and at some point that mortal frailty will be exposed and there will be nothing we can reasonably do about it. To believe otherwise is to reject the nature of creatureliness and buy into an idolatrous vision of medicine.

This raises other questions about the ethics of transplants, such as the assumption that our bodies are mechanisms with interchangeable parts, and the way that current discourse and practice entails the commodification of bodies and their subjection to an autonomous consumerist will.[5] As Campbell notes, this very assumption buys into (so to speak) the market mentality of modern capitalism and so allows for the very possibility of imagining a market in organs.[6] Once the world is imagined in those ways, it becomes next to impossible to argue against such a market – for there is no inherent value in a body and its parts, live or dead, only its value for persons – and that value can only really be measured in monetary terms. But the very fact of thinking

5 See Jeffrey P. Bishop, *The Anticipatory Corpse: Medicine, Power and the Care of the Dying* (Notre Dame, IN: UNDP, 2011), Chs. 3, 5 and 6; Alastair V. Campbell, *The Body in Bioethics* (London: Routledge, 2009); Gerald P. McKenny, *To Relieve the Human Condition: Bioethics, Technology, and the Body* (Albany: University of New York Press, 1997), 184–226.

6 Campbell, *The Body in Bioethics*, 27–53.

in those terms, as Hauerwas might say, discloses a deep-seated corruption of our moral imaginations that cannot and must not be addressed on its own terms. We need to re-imagine the conversation. That, in turn, means thinking more carefully about the nature of bodily existence and the value of it – even after death; the way that our respect for a person's body is an extension of our respect for them; and the way that our practices of dying and death and bereavement and grief reflect an underlying vision of human community. This raises questions about what the practices that surround the 'procurement' of organs for transplant say about our impoverished societies and social imaginations, and the way that the discourses of the transplant industry distort and devalue our understanding of the body, of life in the body, and the leaving of it.

This flows on to questions about the legitimacy of 'brain death' and the validity and application of the 'dead donor rule'. It seems to me that the debate about 'brain death' may not only be an artefact of this technology (and generate artificial categories that serve merely functional ends) but an unhelpful distraction from the kinds of questions we should be asking about death, dying, and how we care for those who are dying (as well as those whose dying is inevitable unless they get an appropriate 'spare part', to put it crassly and with deliberate provocation).[7] There are important questions to ask about the appropriate care of those whose death is inevitable and for whom extended 'curative' treatment might be best seen as extending their dying rather than extending or prolonging their life (to which I will turn in a moment). There are also other, and quite different, questions to ask about how we care for those with end-stage organ failure for whom transplantation provides the only chance of a return to a reasonable level of relational function. Unfortunately, our discussions of 'brain death' and 'organ procurement' have conflated these questions which are quite distinct both in theory and practice; and, more puzzlingly, we haven't noticed that we've done so. Of course, there are important questions to ask about whether 'brain death' is a valid criterion for the death of a person. It is interesting to note how important organ donation has been to questions relating to the definition of death, and problems associated with and

[7] See Bishop, *The Anticipatory Corpse*, 168–222.

proposed solutions to the question of whether death consists in cessation of cardiopulmonary function, or of brain activity, or of higher cortical function, or whether something like organismic dis-integration counts as death.[8] However, framing the question in light of whether someone is/not dead before we 'harvest' their organs already betrays important and questionable metaphysical and moral assumptions. Furthermore, it has already distorted the perspective we have in caring for the person who is dead or dying. They become a 'resource' to be utilized, not a person-in-relationship, someone who needs to be cared for while they are dying, even as we care for those in relationship with them.[9] Once again, important – and deeply rooted – theological and philosophical questions are entailed in these matters. I think it is clear that, whatever we decide about them, philosophy and theology of medicine prompts us to rethink the ethics of transplants.

Reconsidering euthanasia

It also, I believe, prompts us to rethink euthanasia and associated questions of end of life care. Now most discussions of these issues rightly place euthanasia in the broader context of end of life care and the treatment options available to those who are dying.[10] As we have already seen, euthanasia depends on the notion or (often hidden) assumption that medicine exists to enable autonomous individuals to overcome frailty and finitude so as to exercise their freedom. And when it is unable to 'heal' them or alleviate their distress, its role is to facilitate their freely chosen decision to end their life, for suffering is

[8] For a helpful summary of the discussion, see David DeGrazia, The Definition of Death, ed. Edward N. Zalta, *The Stanford Encyclopedia of Philosophy* (Fall 2011 edn) (2011), http://plato.stanford.edu/archives/fall2011/entries/death-definition/ (accessed 19/12/14); see also Nicholas Tonti-Filippini, Religious and Secular Death: A Parting of the Ways, *Bioethics* 26, no. 8 (2012).

[9] Courtney S. Campbell, Harvesting the Living? Separating 'Brain Death' and Organ Transplantation, in *On Moral Medicine: Theological Perspectives in Medical Ethics*, ed. M. Therese Lysaught et al. (Grand Rapids: Eerdmans, 2012).

[10] Although it should be noted that public policy, medical practice and ethical debate now also includes consideration of euthanasia for those with non-terminal conditions, such as mental illness or even, in one tragic instance, unsatisfactory gender reassignment surgery (http://www.dailymail.co.uk/news/article-2440086/Belgian-transsexual-Nathan-Verhelst-44-elects-die-euthanasia-botched-sex-change-operation.html) (accessed 23/07/15). I will limit my discussion to end of life issues, for if euthanasia is not justified in those instances, as I believe to be the case, then it will be even less appropriate for those with non-terminal conditions.

meaningless unless it is voluntarily embraced for some chosen end. If medicine, however, is not a form of technical mastery in service of autonomous wills but a way in which we accept our frailty and by which communities stand in solidarity with their vulnerable members, then these arguments collapse. Indeed, euthanasia comes to be seen as yet another way in which our societies blind themselves to frailty and finitude and abandon those whose vulnerability exposes our delusions, terminating the sufferer as a means of terminating their suffering and hiding it from our a/moral gaze. Indeed, it is a clear expression of the dangers of allowing medicine to be seen as a matter of healing or the alleviation of suffering, for it exposes the way that having reached the end of its healing or ameliorating capacity, medicine withdraws from the field, or implements its final technical solution in the embrace of death.

Re-envisioning medicine as being a matter of caring for vulnerable people requires that we ask what kind of care is appropriate for this dying person; in particular, in what circumstances is it appropriate to reorient our care away from 'cure' and towards other ends? To answer this question, we need to return to the criterion of care I outlined above. When there is no reasonable possibility of a person returning to a reasonable level of relational functioning, then the continued provision of curative therapy is not justified, and so it should be withdrawn or withheld. This does not mean the end of medical care for this person, for when life-prolonging therapy is withdrawn or withheld, it is time for the provision of active and intensive *palliative* care. Palliative care aims at delivering the care this person needs to live as well as they can while dying: that is, to maximize their relational functioning even though there is no prospect of a return to health. Thus, the *goal* of this practice is not that person's death, but the provision of the appropriate kind of therapy for them at this stage of their living or dying. We are, I believe, required to provide such care to dying people, even though it will not lead to their healing or improved health. Palliative care, indeed, should be included as part of basic health care to which we are entitled as one of our sustenance rights, for it is needed for the reasonable relational functioning of the dying. Indeed, it is required of a society if it is to be just and loving towards those of its members who are dying, who, despite their lack of present or future social utility, are still a part of the web of relationships and institutions which constitutes a society. It also allows us to turn our gaze towards rather than away from our inherent vulnerability and is a clear expression of our solidarity with, rather than abandonment of, fellow humans at the end of their lives.[11]

Majority world medicine, scarcity and medicine as a moral practice

In many respects, the key questions relating to the role of medicine in conditions of scarcity flow naturally from the preceding discussion. If, as I have argued, we have medical sustenance rights, then those rights apply to people wherever they happen to be, in whatever circumstances they happen to live. The precise form and content of what is provided to satisfy those entitlements, however, are situational. That is to say, the basic health care to which everyone is entitled is likely to take different forms in different contexts. While basic medical care in Western contexts comprises, roughly, those services provided by and which cluster around a good general practice, even if the same rough criterion were to apply in, say, Sierra Leone or rural Nepal, quite different services would be provided. This is partly because of the different levels of general social services available in those contexts, partly because of the different needs of people in them. Nutritional advice in Australia, for instance, is most likely going to focus on calorie restriction, a balanced diet and weight loss; in Sierra Leone or Nepal, it is most likely going to focus on sanitation, a balanced diet and treating malnutrition and dietary deficiencies. A GP in suburban Australia will be able to refer their patient for sophisticated investigations in the immediate vicinity; in rural Australia, such services may be at the end of a four-hour drive. A local health worker in rural Nepal is unlikely to be able to refer their patient for any sophisticated investigations as they may be a number of days' journey away, the patient cannot afford the time and the travel, and would not be able to pay for them even if they were available. A more basic level of medical treatment is

11 See also Lisa Sowle Cahill, *Theological Bioethics: Participation, Justice, Change* (Washington, DC: Georgetown University Press, 2005), 102–130; Jeffrey P. Bishop, The Hard Work of Dying, http://www.abc.net.au/religion/articles/2014/07/15/4046423.htm (accessed 16/04/15).

appropriate.[12] Nonetheless, all people are entitled to access to such services. We ought to be scandalized that even where the government notionally provides, say, rural health clinics, they are often under-resourced, incompetently run, and under- or even un-staffed. A Christian understanding of medicine sees this as simply unacceptable.

However, it also needs to remember that medicine is a large and complex social practice that is located in and sustained by broader social arrangements. Indeed, we must remember that any entitlement to medical services is connected to a broader set of sustenance rights, all of which must be provided by a society to its members (whether by centralized governmental control or market forces is irrelevant). And so, if we are concerned about the provision of medical sustenance rights, we need to be equally concerned about the provision of the others. This, of course, makes practical sense as well. For only in a stable society and a functional economy are the systems of supply of resources, dependable rule of law, education, and so on going to permit the development of the training and technical facilities needed to sustain any level of medical care, or the means of access and basic trust that allow for a sense of being able to depend reliably on medical services. Clearly, an integrated vision for social transformation is needed; indeed, if observations about the importance to the health and well-being of communities of non-medical services such as clean water, sanitation, education, basic social stability, and so forth are true, and our concern for adequate medical services arises out of a concern for *shalom*, for human flourishing, then such a broad vision of social transformation is entailed in any legitimate picture of medicine in our global context. This brings to bear questions of justice within and between nations and economies, power and its mis/use in global and local political institutions, patterns of trade and economic and educational disparities – and the bitterly ironic fact that, despite the scattered generosity of Western nations, the net flow of money and expertise (including trained doctors and nurses) is *from* the majority world *to* the West. Once again, medicine is not quarantined from bigger questions of justice and our responsibilities in a globalized world: any legitimate reflection

12 For a brief, focused discussion on these questions, see Sloane, Painful Justice. See also Robin Attfield, The Global Distribution of Health Care Resources, *Journal of Medical Ethics* 16 (1990).

on Christianity and medicine needs to come to terms with these broader questions; so, too, must our practice.[13] Costly engagement in risky contexts, such as has been typical of Christian medical mission (and also the recent work of *MSF*), is an appropriate, even necessary, expression of such a vision.

This raises questions, of course, about what is then owed to the people who take such risks and pay such prices in caring for vulnerable people in contexts such as rural Nepal or plague-ridden Sierra Leone.[14] First, let me make it plain, in case it isn't already: it is not only appropriate for some doctors to take such risks in caring for vulnerable people in situations of want, whether in their own country or not; it is incumbent on us as Christians and as professionals that some of us do so. A Christian vision of a properly functioning community is one in which all its members are able to flourish: anything less than that falls far short of the goal of *shalom* that is God's creational and redemptive purpose for humans in community. But a Christian social vision cannot be bound by national borders, as if the country on our passport establishes the limits of our vision. Flourishing is God's intention for *all* human beings, for *every* human community. We are all diminished whenever we accept less than this for any of God's children. And so, while not all of us are called into medical mission (or aid and development work), some of us are. This is not a selfish expression of a privatized sense of God's calling on an individual soul; it is a response to God's call on our communities, and the ways in which they ought to be shaped in response to God's character and purpose. Embracing such a call is rarely 'heroic'; it is too long term for heroism. It entails the hard grind of language learning, gaining cultural sensitivity, context-specific training, enduring, small-scale sacrifices, and the cost to normal career progression. This is hardly heroic. But it may be saintly.

Now, if we see it as an outworking of a vision of life-in-community rather than just a response to a private heavenly voice, then we who do not go have

13 For general theological reflections on these questions, see my discussion in: Andrew Sloane, The Old Testament and Christian Social Engagement, in *Another Way to Love: Christian Social Reform and Global Poverty*, ed. Tim Costello and Rod Yule (Brunswick East: Acorn, 2009); Love and Justice in International Frame, *Case* 22 (2010); Justifying Advocacy: A Biblical and Theological Rationale for Speaking the Truth to Power on Behalf of the Vulnerable, *Evangelical Review of Theology* 36, no. 2 (2012).

14 These are questions that Christians have been asking – and answering – since the beginning of the Christian movement. See the discussion of Christian responses to plague in Roman cities in Rodney Stark, *The Rise of Christianity* (New York: HarperCollins, 1996), 73–94.

responsibilities to those who do. They are our representatives, signs to the world that God and God's people actually care about the love and fidelity and justice that we say are our ideals. We can no more send them and forget them than the early apostolic churches could send and forget their missionaries. We are called into solidarity with those who express our solidarity with vulnerable people in difficult and dangerous circumstances. And so when those carers become at risk, when they fall prey to the conditions they seek to address, then it is our responsibility to care for them as if they were our own – as indeed, they are. While it may seem extravagant, costly medical evacuation to tertiary medical centres simply gives these people access to the services they would otherwise have had at home. These services may be medical mercies, but when they are provided by a community, they need to be provided equitably and justly. Australia's famous Flying Doctor service is an expression of that vision within the broad and extensive borders of our sparsely settled country. Medical evacuation is an extension of that beyond our borders, stretching the boundaries of our responsibilities as far as those who extend the margins of our care have gone. So, while a willingness to risk life and well-being in caring for others is controversial and has been rejected by people from Galen to contemporary bioethicists, it has typified Christian care for the sick from earliest times.[15] Furthermore, it expresses something important about medicine and the cultural imagination that makes an enterprise like modern medicine possible.[16]

Concluding pedagogical reflections

As I bring this book to a close, I would like to gather a few of the dangling threads of argument and weave them into suggestions about how Christian reflections on the nature and goals of medicine might inform medical education. If medicine is an expression of a community's solidarity with those

[15] For the contrast between Galen's and early Christian responses, see Stark, *The Rise of Christianity*, 85–86; for the contemporary discussion, see http://www.theweek.co.uk/world-news/ebola/60994/ebola-should-doctors-be-forced-to-treat-infected-patients (accessed 17/04/15).

[16] For the claim that such care for the weak is, in fact, a product of the Christianizing of Western culture, see David Bentley Hart, *Atheist Delusions: The Christian Revolution and its Fashionable Enemies* (New Haven: Yale University Press, 2009), esp. Part Three.

whose vulnerability is exposed by a disruption to their physical or psychological integrity, and if its goal is to express appropriate forms of care for frail, embodied creatures, how might this impact the way we train doctors? Elsewhere, I have mentioned how it ought to prompt concern for the development of moral qualities as well as the technical and relational expertise required, which has been the focus of most medical education.[17] I think those comments still stand; but now, I want to turn my attention to questions of medical epistemology, the internal goods of medicine and their relationship to other goals that may distort or corrupt the practice of medicine, and the expectations people in the West have about what medicine can deliver.

As I discussed earlier, medicine's knowledge is fundamentally embodied. In clinical medicine, we are 'knowing bodies'. That is to say, the aim of our practices of inquiry is to understand what is going on in the some-body before us; to get to grips with that disruption to their ability to function in the world (or their – or our – fears about such disruption) that prompt them to see us as doctors. And the primary way in which we come to understand what is going on is by using our own bodies to understand theirs: to listen carefully to their stories so as to discern both what matters to them and how we might appraise that medically; to use touch and hearing and our other senses – direct and mediated through such instruments as stethoscopes and thermometers – to discover what's going on beneath the surface. Such basic history-taking and clinical examination takes time to do, and time to master, but it is fundamental to clinical practice. Indeed, it is, I would suggest, one of the ways that a good doctor benefits their patient. A patient feels heard – and touched – and so no longer isolated in their illness. An undue focus on investigations both detracts from the human element of the clinical encounter, and wrongly understands the nature and goals of medical knowledge. There seems to be a tendency to devalue basic history-taking and physical examination in medical education in favour of 'objective' and measurable investigations.[18] Inculcating a better understanding of the nature and goals of medicine might contribute to a

17 Sloane, Christianity and the Transformation of Medicine, 94–95.

18 This is partly, I suspect, due to the increasingly litigious nature of the doctor–patient relationship and the growing practice of (medico-legal) defensive medicine; it is also, I think, the result of an over-valuing of hard empirical data and a loss of trust in personal judgement. I am grateful to Dr Megan Best for a conversation (13/05/2013) that helped stimulate these reflections.

return to a focus on engaging with persons in diagnosis and treatment, and in this regard medical education plays a crucial role.

It might also allow for a better integration of 'medical humanities' into the curriculum.[19] It is interesting to note that, for all its scientific rigour, medicine occupies a strange place in the university. It doesn't so much occupy the borders or no man's land between the humanities and the physical sciences as it squarely occupies territory deep within the borders of both sets of disciplines. For it seeks to know and care for embodied persons; and that care entails understanding and dealing with the physical phenomena that beset us and the personal and social and spiritual issues that are thrown up by them (and cause or contribute to them). Moreover, while basic sciences such as biology are fundamental to the body of knowledge that informs clinical medical practice, medicine is itself a practical enterprise (and activity of practical wisdom, perhaps) rather than a basic science. This means it is different to the knowledge of both EBM and bench science and the kinds of certainty that they require for statistical analysis of populations or basic science, respectively. This, too, means that a focus on hard data from investigations rather than clinical judgement misunderstands and distorts the nature of medical knowledge. Furthermore, epistemologically there are justifiable limits of the extent and kind of knowledge medicine ought to have. For (clinical) medical knowledge is praxis-oriented theory and so is justified in as much as it helps achieve certain ends, notably, to provide appropriate care for people. Requiring a greater level of certainty than is needed for the effective treatment of a patient would not only be inappropriate patient care, it is likely to interfere with broader social obligations regarding the use of time, expertise, resources, and so forth. Helping students understand the nature, justification and limits of medical knowledge would help rehumanize them and their care as well as enabling better use of available resources. It also allows them to integrate an understanding of medical knowledge into a broader understanding of medicine.

[19] See James Arthur et al., Virtuous Medical Practice (The Jubilee Centre for Character and Virtues, University of Birmingham, 2015); Daniel Callahan, Medical Education and the Goals of Medicine, *Medical Teacher* 20, no. 2 (1998); Jane Macnaughton, Medical Humanities' Challenge to Medicine, *Journal of Evaluation in Clinical Practice* 17, no. 5 (2011); David Misselbrook, *Thinking about Patients* (Plymouth: Petroc, 2001).

That broader understanding of medicine also requires that we integrate notions of medicine as an inherently moral *profession* into our training of doctors. While medical paternalism has been justifiably critiqued, the notion of medicine as a social practice with its own ends and as entailing the responsible exercise of that power entrusted by society and patients to doctors requires some notion of medicine as a moral profession. The loss of this understanding has contributed to the increasing commodification of medicine, as it has become reduced to the application of technical mastery to the enhancing of consumers' personal projects. Refocusing medical education on medicine as a practice would mean sustained reflection on the goods that are internal to it as a practice, and the way that the replacement of them by external goods, such as money or social utility, inevitably leads to its corruption. Moreover, it would encourage doctors (and those who train them) to consider how treating medicine as a commodity recognizes neither the way such views are complicit in late modern industrial capitalism nor the way that medicine deals with the kind of vulnerability that threatens a person's engagement in the market and other such 'autonomous' projects. Of course, it also requires a reconfiguring of what medicine can and cannot do for us, and how those expectations arise out of larger understandings of the world and our role in it. Again, philosophical reflection on medicine as a practice would enrich both medical education and the practice of those so shaped.

Now, it's plain that I have given neither an exhaustive account of medicine, nor a comprehensive answer to many of the questions raised in this book. And I suspect that what I have said will not persuade everyone. Indeed, it's likely that, while you have found answers to important questions, you may finish the book with more questions than you had when you started. That wouldn't surprise me: it is not unheard of for students to say something similar at the end of my classes. But then, I'm OK with that: my job is, after all, not (just) to provide answers, but to get people to *think*, and think Christianly. I believe I have presented a philosophy and theology of medicine that both articulates a Christian view of the world and illuminates the nature and practice of medicine. I tried to think Christianly about this significant and complex practice. Perhaps more importantly, I hope it has prompted you to do likewise, whether you agree with me or not.

Bibliography

Anderson, Bernhard W., and Steven Bishop. *Contours of Old Testament Theology*. Minneapolis: Fortress, 1998.

Arthur, James, Kristján Kristjánsson, Hywel Thomas, Ben Kotzee, Agnieszka Ignatowicz, and Tian Qiu. Virtuous Medical Practice, 1–35: The Jubilee Centre for Character and Virtues, University of Birmingham, 2015.

Atkinson, D. J. Causing Death and Allowing to Die. *Tyndale Bulletin* 34 (1983): 201–228.

Attfield, Robin. The Global Distribution of Health Care Resources. *Journal of Medical Ethics* 16 (1990): 153–156.

Badham, Paul. Should Christians Accept the Validity of Voluntary Euthanasia?. *Studies in Christian Ethics* 8, no. 2 (1995): 1–12.

Banks, Sarah, and Ann Gallagher. *Ethics in Professional Life: Virtues for Health and Social Care*. Basingstoke: Palgrave Macmillan, 2009.

Barr, James. *The Concept of Biblical Theology: An Old Testament Perspective*. London: SCM, 1999.

Barr, James. *The Semantics of Biblical Language*. Oxford: Oxford University Press, 1961.

Barth, Karl. *The Doctrine of Creation: Church Dogmatics*, 4 vols London: T&T Clark, 1956–1975.

Bartholomew, Craig G., and Michael W. Goheen. *The Drama of Scripture: Finding Our Place in the Biblical Story*. Grand Rapids: Baker Academic, 2004.

Baum, Fran. *The New Public Health*. 3rd edn. South Melbourne: Oxford University Press, 2008.

Beauchamp, Tom L. The 'Four Principles' Approach. In *Meaning and Medicine: A Reader in the Philosophy of Health Care*, edited by J. L. Nelson and H. L. Nelson, 147–155. New York: Routledge, 1999.

Beauchamp, Tom L., and James F. Childress. *Principles of Biomedical Ethics*, 7th edn. Oxford: Oxford University Press, 2008.

Beavis, Mary Ann. *Mark*. Grand Rapids: Baker, 2011.

Best, Megan. *Fearfully and Wonderfully Made: Ethics and the Beginning of Human Life*. Sydney: Matthias Media, 2012.

Bishop, Jeffrey P. *The Anticipatory Corpse: Medicine, Power and the Care of the Dying*. Notre Dame, IN: UNDP, 2011.

Bishop, Jeffrey P. Biopsychosociospiritual Medicine and Other Political Schemes. *Christian Bioethics: Non-Ecumenical Studies in Medical Morality* 15, no. 3 (2009): 254–276.

Bishop, Jeffrey P. Foucauldian Diagnostics: Space, Time, and the Metaphysics of Medicine. *Journal of Medicine and Philosophy* 34, no. 4 (2009): 328–349.

Bishop, Jeffrey P. The Hard Work of Dying. http://www.abc.net.au/religion/articles/2014/07/15/4046423.htm.

Black, C. Clifton. *Mark*. Nashville: Abingdon, 2011.

Bloesch, Donald G. *Freedom for Obedience: Evangelical Ethics in Contemporary Times.* San Francisco: Harper & Row, 1987.

Bluhm, Robyn, and Kirstin Borgerson. Evidence-Based Medicine. In *Philosophy of Medicine*, edited by Fred Gifford, 203–238. Amsterdam: Elsevier, 2011.

Bonhoeffer, Dietrich. *Ethics*. Translated by N. H. Smith. London: SCM, 1955.

Boorse, Christopher. Concepts of Health and Disease. In *Philosophy of Medicine*, edited by Fred Gifford, 13–64. Amsterdam: Elsevier, 2011.

Boorse, Christopher. On the Distinction between Disease and Illness. In *Meaning and Medicine: A Reader in the Philosophy of Health Care*, edited by J. L. Nelson and H. L. Nelson, 16–27. New York: Routledge, 1999.

Bratton, Susan Power. *Six Billion and More: Human Population Regulation and Christian Ethics*. Louisville: Westminster / John Knox, 1992.

Brueggemann, Walter. Biblical Theology Appropriately Postmodern. *Biblical Theology Bulletin* 27 (1997): 4–9.

Brueggemann, Walter. *Theology of the Old Testament: Testimony, Dispute, Advocacy.* Minneapolis: Fortress, 1997.

Cahill, Lisa Sowle. Theologians and Bioethicists: Some History and a Proposal. In *On Moral Medicine: Theological Perspectives in Medical Ethics*, edited by M. Therese Lysaught, Joseph J. Kotva, Jr, Stephen E. Lammers, and Allen Verhey, 60–76. Grand Rapids: Eerdmans, 2012.

Cahill, Lisa Sowle. *Theological Bioethics: Participation, Justice, Change*. Washington, DC: Georgetown University Press, 2005.

Callahan, Daniel. Medical Education and the Goals of Medicine. *Medical Teacher* 20, no. 2 (1998): 85–86.

Cameron, Nigel M. de S. The Christian Stake in Bioethics: The State of the Question. In *Bioethics and the Future of Medicine: A Christian Appraisal*, edited by John F. Kilner, Nigel M. de S. Cameron, and David L. Schiedermayer, 3–13. Carlisle: Paternoster, 1995.

Cameron, Nigel M. de S. *The New Medicine: The Revolution in Technology and Ethics.* London: Hodder & Stoughton, 1991.

Campbell, Alastair V. *The Body in Bioethics*. London: Routledge, 2009.

Campbell, Courtney S. Harvesting the Living? Separating 'Brain Death' and Organ Transplantation. In *On Moral Medicine: Theological Perspectives in Medical Ethics*, edited by M. Therese Lysaught, Joseph J. Kotva, Jr, Stephen E. Lammers, and Allen Verhey, 437–444. Grand Rapids: Eerdmans, 2012.

Carey, William. *An Enquiry into the Obligations of Christians, to Use Means for the Conversion of the Heathens*. Leicester: Ann Ireland, 1792. http://www.wmcarey.edu/carey/enquiry/anenquiry.pdf.

Carson, Don. Current Issues in Biblical Theology: A New Testament Perspective. *Bulletin for Biblical Research* 5 (1995): 17–41.

Clouser, K. Danner, and Bernard Gert. A Critique of Principlism. In *Meaning and Medicine: A Reader in the Philosophy of Health Care*, edited by J. L. Nelson and H. L. Nelson, 156–166. New York: Routledge, 1999.

Cole, R. Alan. *Mark: An Introduction and Commentary*. Nottingham: IVP, 1989.

Cooper, Denise Anne. The Doctor as Moral Agent, with Reference to the Distinction between Killing and 'Letting Die'. PhD, The University of Melbourne, 2007.

Daniels, Norman. A Lifespan Approach to Health Care. In *Bioethics: An Anthology*, edited by Helga Kuhse and Peter Singer, 465–474. Oxford: Blackwell, 2006.

DeGrazia, David. The Definition of Death. In *The Stanford Encyclopedia of Philosophy* (Fall 2011 edn), edited by Edward N. Zalta, 2011. http://plato.stanford.edu/archives/fall2011/entries/death-definition.

Delamothe, Tony, Rosamund Snow, and Fiona Godlee. Why the Assisted Dying Bill Should Become Law in England and Wales. *British Medical Journal* 349 (2014).

Dempster, Stephen G. *Dominion and Dynasty: A Theology of the Hebrew Bible*. Leicester: Apollos, 2003.

Donahue, John R., and Daniel J. Harrington. *The Gospel of Mark*. Collegeville: Liturgical Press, 2002.

Doornbos, Mary Molewyk, Ruth E. Groenhout, and Kendra G. Hotz. *Transforming Care: A Christian Vision of Nursing Practice*. Grand Rapids: Eerdmans, 2005.

Dworkin, Gerald. Physician-Assisted Death: The State of the Debate. In *The Oxford Handbook of Bioethics*, edited by Bonnie Steinbock, 375–392. Oxford: Oxford University Press, 2007.

Eddy, David M. Evidence-Based Medicine: A Unified Approach. *Health Affairs* 24, no. 1 (2005): 9–17.

Eddy, David M. The Origins of Evidence-Based Medicine – a Personal Perspective. *Virtual Mentor* 13, no. 1 (2011): 55–60.

Eiesland, Nancy L. Encountering the Disabled God. In *On Moral Medicine: Theological Perspectives in Medical Ethics*, edited by M. Therese Lysaught, Joseph J. Kotva, Jr, Stephen E. Lammers, and Allen Verhey, 587–589. Grand Rapids: Eerdmans, 2012.

Engel, George L. The Need for a New Medical Model: A Challenge for Biomedicine. *Family Systems Medicine* 10, no. 3 (Fall 1992): 317–331.

Engelhardt, H. Tristram, Jr. Christian Bioethics after Christendom: Living in a Secular Fundamentalist Polity and Culture. *Christian Bioethics: Non-Ecumenical Studies in Medical Morality* 17, no. 1 (01// 2011): 64–95.

Engelhardt, H. Tristram, Jr. Bioethics at the End of the Millennium: Fashioning Health Care Policy in the Absence of a Moral Consensus. In *Ethical Issues in Health Care on the Frontiers of the Twenty-First Century*, edited by Stephen Wear, James J. Bono, Gerald Logue, and Adrianne McEvoy, 1–16. Dordrecht: Kluwer, 2000.

Engelhardt, H. Tristram, Jr. The Disease of Masturbation: Values and the Concept of Disease. In *Meaning and Medicine: A Reader in the Philosophy of Health Care*, edited by H. L. Nelson and J. L. Nelson, 5–15. New York: Routledge, 1999.

Engelhardt, H. Tristram, Jr. Global Bioethics, Theology, and Human Genetic Engineering: The Challenge of Refashioning Human Nature in the Face of Moral and Religious Pluralism. In *Genethics and Religion*, edited by G. Phleiderer, G. Brahier, and K. Lindpaintner. Basel: Krager, 2010.

Fackre, Gabriel. *The Christian Story*, 3rd edn. Grand Rapids: Eerdmans, 1996.

Foucault, Michel. *The Birth of the Clinic: An Archaeology of Medical Perception*. New York: Vintage, 1963, 1994.

Fountain, Daniel E. *Health, the Bible and the Church*. Wheaton: Billy Graham Centre, 1989.

France, R. T. *The Gospel of Mark: A Commentary on the Greek Text*. Grand Rapids: Eerdmans, 2002.

Gawande, Atul. *Being Mortal: Medicine and What Matters in the End*. New York: Metropolitan Books, 2014.

Gergel, Tania L. Medicine and the Individual: Is Phenomenology the Answer?. *Journal of Evaluation in Clinical Practice* 18, no. 5 (2012): 1102–1109.

Gifford, Fred (ed.). *Philosophy of Medicine*, Handbook of the Philosophy of Science. Amsterdam: Elsevier, 2011.

Guelich, Robert A. *Mark 1–8:26*. Dallas: Word, 1989.

Gustafson, James M. Theology Confronts Technology and the Life Sciences. *Commonweal* 105 (1978): 386–392.

Hall, Daniel E., Harold G. Koenig, and Keith G. Meador. Conceptualizing 'Religion': How Language Shapes and Constrains Knowledge in the Study of Religion and Health. *Perspectives in Biology and Medicine* 47, no. 3 (2004): 386–401.

Hare, John. *God's Call: Moral Realism, God's Commands, and Human Autonomy*. Grand Rapids: Eerdmans, 2001.

Hare, John. *Why Bother Being Good? The Place of God in the Moral Life*. Downers Grove: IVP, 2002.

Hare, R. M. Health. *Journal of Medical Ethics* 12, no. 4 (1986): 174–181.

Hart, David Bentley. *Atheist Delusions: The Christian Revolution and Its Fashionable Enemies*. New Haven: Yale University Press, 2009.

Hart, David Bentley. God or Nothingness. In *I Am the Lord Your God: Christian Reflections on the Ten Commandments*, edited by Carl E. Braaten and Christopher R. Seitz, 55–76. Grand Rapids: Eerdmans, 2005.

Hastings Center. Specifying the Goals of Medicine. *Hastings Center Report* 26, no. 6 (1996): S9.

Hauerwas, Stanley. *Naming the Silences: God, Medicine, and the Problem of Suffering*. Grand Rapids: Eerdmans, 1990.

Hauerwas, Stanley. *The Peaceable Kingdom: A Primer in Christian Ethics*. London: SCM, 1983.

Hauerwas, Stanley. *Suffering Presence: Theological Reflections on Medicine, the Mentally Handicapped, and the Church*. Edinburgh: T&T Clark, 1986.

Hauerwas, Stanley. The End of American Protestantism. http://www.abc.net.au/religion/articles/2013/07/02/3794561.htm.

Hays, Richard. *The Moral Vision of the New Testament: A Contemporary Introduction to New Testament Ethics*. New York: HarperCollins, 1996.

Henry, Stephen G. Polanyi's Tacit Knowing and the Relevance of Epistemology to Clinical Medicine. *Journal of Evaluation in Clinical Practice* 16, no. 2 (2010): 292–297.

Hesslow, Germund. Do We Need a Concept of Disease?. *Theoretical Medicine* 14 (1993): 1–14.

Hotz, Kendra G., and Matthew T. Mathews. *Dust and Breath: Faith, Health, and Why the Church Should Care about Both*. Grand Rapids: Eerdmans, 2012.

Huber, Machteld, J. André Knotterus, Lawrence Green, Henriëtte van der Horst, Alejandro R. Jadad, Daan Kromhout, Brian Leonard, et al. How Should We Define Health?, *British Medical Journal* 343 (2011): 1–3.

Hunter, James Davison. *To Change the World: The Irony, Tragedy, and Possibility of Christianity in the Late Modern World*. Oxford: Oxford University Press, 2010.

Hurtado, Larry W. *Mark*. Peabody: Hendrickson, 1989.

Jotterand, Fabrice. The Hippocratic Oath and Contemporary Medicine: Dialectic between Past Ideals and Present Reality?. *Journal of Medicine and Philosophy* 30 (2005): 107–128.

Juel, Donald H. *Mark*. Minneapolis: Augsburg, 1990.

Kant, Immanuel. *Critique of Pure Reason*. London: G. Bell, 1781, 1922.

Keenan, James F. The Case for Physician-Assisted Suicide?. In *On Moral Medicine: Theological Perspectives in Medical Ethics*, edited by M. Therese Lysaught, Joseph J. Kotva, Jr, Stephen E. Lammers, and Allen Verhey, 1085–1088. Grand Rapids: Eerdmans, 2012.

Khushf, George. Illness, the Problem of Evil, and the Analogical Structure of Healing: On the Difference Christianity Makes in Bioethics. *Christian Bioethics* 1, no. 1 (1995): 102–120.

Kotva, Joseph J., Jr. The Christian Pastor's Role in Medical Ethics: In the Pew and at the Bedside. In *On Moral Medicine: Theological Perspectives in Medical Ethics*, edited by M. Therese Lysaught, Joseph J. Kotva, Jr, Stephen E. Lammers, and Allen Verhey, 272–282. Grand Rapids: Eerdmans, 2012.

Kotva, Joseph J., Jr. Hospital Chaplaincy as Apapeic Intervention. In *On Moral Medicine: Theological Perspectives in Medical Ethics*, edited by M. Therese Lysaught, Joseph J. Kotva, Jr, Stephen E. Lammers, and Allen Verhey, 260–268. Grand Rapids: Eerdmans, 2012.

Kraftchick, Steven J., Jr, Charles D. Myers, and Ben C. Ollenburger (eds.). *Biblical Theology: Problems and Perspectives*. Nashville: Abingdon, 1995.

Kuhn, Thomas. *The Structure of Scientific Revolutions*, 2nd edn. Chicago: University of Chicago Press, 1970.

Kung, Hans. A Dignified Dying. In *On Moral Medicine: Theological Perspectives in Medical Ethics*, edited by M. Therese Lysaught, Joseph J. Kotva, Jr, Stephen E. Lammers, and Allen Verhey, 1090–1097. Grand Rapids: Eerdmans, 2012.

Lang, Eddy. The Why and the How of Evidence-Based Medicine. *McGill Journal of Medicine* 8 (2004): 90–94.

Lickiss, N. Euthanasia from the Perspective of a Palliative Care Consultant. Paper presented at the Proceedings of Conference on Active Voluntary Euthanasia, Monash University Centre for Human Bioethics, 15 November 1993.

Lindbeck, George. *The Nature of Doctrine: Religion and Theology in a Postliberal Age*. Phildelphia: Westminster, 1984.

Little, Miles. 'Better Than Numbers . . .': A Gentle Critique of Evidence-Based Medicine. In *Restoring Humane Values to Medicine: A Miles Little Reader*, edited by Ian Kerridge, Christopher Jordens, and Emma-Jane Sayers, 103–129. Sydney: Desert Pea, 2003.

Little, Miles, and Stephen Leeder. Logic, Hermeneutics and Informed Consent. In *Restoring Humane Values to Medicine: A Miles Little Reader*, edited by Ian Kerridge, Christopher Jordens, and Emma-Jane Sayers, 151–165. Sydney: Desert Pea, 2003.

Long, D. Stephen. The Language of Death: Theology and Economics in Conflict. In *On Moral Medicine: Theological Perspectives in Medical Ethics*, edited by

M. Therese Lysaught, Joseph J. Kotva, Jr, Stephen E. Lammers, and Allen Verhey, 551–560. Grand Rapids: Eerdmans, 2012.

Long, W. Meredith. *Health, Healing and God's Kingdom*. Oxford: Regnum, 2000.

Loughlin, Michael, Robyn Bluhm, Jonathan Fuller, Stephen Buetow, Ross E. G. Upshur, Kirstin Borgerson, Maya J. Goldenberg, and Elselijn Kingma. Philosophy, Medicine and Health Care – Where We Have Come From and Where We Are Going. *Journal of Evaluation in Clinical Practice* 20 (2014): 902–907.

Lysaught, M. Therese, Joseph J. Kotva, Jr, Stephen E. Lammers, and Allen Verhey (eds.). *On Moral Medicine: Theological Perspectives in Medical Ethics*, 3rd edn. Grand Rapids: Eerdmans, 2012.

MacIntyre, Alasdair. *After Virtue: A Study in Moral Theory*. 2nd edn. Notre Dame: University of Notre Dame Press, 1984.

MacIntyre, Alasdair. *Dependent Rational Animals: Why Human Beings Need the Virtues*. London: Duckworth, 1999.

MacIntyre, Alasdair. *Whose Justice? Which Rationality?* London: Duckworth, 1987.

Macnaughton, Jane. Medical Humanities' Challenge to Medicine. *Journal of Evaluation in Clinical Practice* 17, no. 5 (2011): 927–932.

Marcus, Joel. *Mark 1–8: A New Translation with Introduction and Commentary*. Garden City: Doubleday, 2000.

Mathúna, Dónal P. Spirituality and Alternative Medicine. In *Cutting-Edge Bioethics: A Christian Exploration of Technologies and Trends*, edited by John F. Kilner, C. Christopher Hook, and Diann B. Uustal, 116–130. Grand Rapids: Eerdmans, 2002.

May, William F. Money and the Medical Profession. *Kennedy Institute of Ethics Journal* 7, no. 1 (1997): 1–13.

McKenny, Gerald P. Bioethics, the Body, and the Legacy of Bacon. In *On Moral Medicine: Theological Perspectives in Medical Ethics*, edited by M. Therese Lysaught, Joseph J. Kotva, Jr, Stephen E. Lammers, and Allen Verhey, 398–409. Grand Rapids: Eerdmans, 2012.

McKenny, Gerald P. *To Relieve the Human Condition: Bioethics, Technology, and the Body*. Albany: University of New York Press, 1997.

Meilaender, Gilbert. *Bioethics: A Primer for Christians*, 3rd edn. Grand Rapids: Eerdmans, 2013.

Meilaender, Gilbert. *Body, Soul, and Bioethics*. Notre Dame: UNDP, 1995.

Messer, Neil G. *Flourishing: Health, Disease, and Bioethics in Theological Perspective*. Grand Rapids: Eerdmans, 2013.

Messer, Neil G. Toward a Theological Understanding of Health and Disease. *Journal of the Society of Christian Ethics* 31, no. 1 (2011): 161–178.

Meulen, Ruud H. J. ter. The Lost Voice: How Libertarianism and Consumerism Obliterate the Need for a Relational Ethics in the National Health Care Service. *Christian Bioethics* 14, no. 1 (2008): 78–94.

Misselbrook, David. *Thinking about Patients.* Plymouth: Petroc, 2001.

Mordacci, Roberto, and Richard Sobel. Health: A Comprehensive Concept. In *Health, Disease, and Illness: Concepts in Medicine*, edited by Arthur L. Caplan, James J. McCartney, and Dominic A. Sisti, 104–109. Washington, DC: Georgetown University Press, 2004.

Moreland, J. P. James Rachels and the Active Euthanasia Debate. *Journal of the Evangelical Theological Society* 31, no. 1 (1988): 81–90.

Morris, John F. Health Care Reform. In *Medicine, Health Care, and Ethics: Catholic Voices*, edited by John F. Morris, 301–308. Washington, DC: Catholic University of America Press, 2007.

Moss, Alvin H., and Mark Siegler. Should Alcoholics Compete Equally for Liver Transplantation?. In *Bioethics: An Anthology*, edited by Helga Kuhse and Peter Singer, 421–427. Oxford: Blackwell, 2006.

Murphy, Dominic. Concepts of Disease and Health. In *The Stanford Encyclopedia of Philosophy* (Summer 2009 edn), edited by Edward N. Zalta, 2009. http://plato.stanford.edu/archives/sum2009/entries/health-disease/.

Nouwen, Henri J. M. *Adam: God's Beloved*. Maryknoll, NY: Orbis, 1997.

O'Donovan, Oliver. *Resurrection and Moral Order: An Outline for Evangelical Ethics*, 2nd edn. Grand Rapids: Eerdmans, 1994.

Pate, C. Marvin, J. Scott Duvall, J. Daniel Hays, E. Randolph Richards, Jr, W. Dennis Tucker, and Preben Vang. *The Story of Israel: A Biblical Theology*. Leicester, UK: Apollos, 2004.

Pellegrino, Edmund D. The Commodification of Medical and Health Care: The Moral Consequences of a Paradigm Shift from a Professional to a Market Ethic. In *The Philosophy of Medicine Reborn: A Pellegrino Reader*, edited by H. Tristram Englehardt, Jr, and Fabrice Jotterand, 101–126. Notre Dame: UNDP, 2008.

Pellegrino, Edmund D. Humanistic Basis of Professional Ethics. In *The Philosophy of Medicine Reborn: A Pellegrino Reader*, edited by H. Tristram Englehardt, Jr, and Fabrice Jotterand, 87–100. Notre Dame: UNDP, 2008.

Pellegrino, Edmund D. The Internal Morality of Clinical Medicine: A Paradigm for the Ethics of the Helping and Healing Professions. In *The Philosophy of Medicine Reborn: A Pellegrino Reader*, edited by H. Tristram Englehardt, Jr, and Fabrice Jotterand, 62–84. Notre Dame: UNDP, 2008.

Pellegrino, Edmund D. Medicine Today: Its Identity, Its Role, and the Role of Physicians. In *The Philosophy of Medicine Reborn: A Pellegrino Reader*, edited by

H. Tristram Englehardt, Jr, and Fabrice Jotterand, 127–146. Notre Dame: UNDP, 2008.

Pellegrino, Edmund D. Philosophy of Medicine: Should It Be Teleologically or Socially Constructed?. In *The Philosophy of Medicine Reborn: A Pellegrino Reader*, edited by H. Tristram Englehardt, Jr, and Fabrice Jotterand, 49–61. Notre Dame: UNDP, 2008.

Pellegrino, Edmund D. What the Philosophy *of* Medicine *Is*. In *The Philosophy of Medicine Reborn: A Pellegrino Reader*, edited by H. Tristram Englehardt, Jr, and Fabrice Jotterand, 23–48. Notre Dame: UNDP, 2008.

Pellegrino, Edmund D., and David C. Thomasma. *The Christian Virtues in Medical Practice*. Washington, DC: Georgetown University Press, 1996.

Pellegrino, Edmund D., and David C. Thomasma. *Helping and Healing: Religious Commitment in Health Care*. Washington, DC: Georgetown University Press, 1997.

Peterson, Alan, and Robin Bunton (eds.). *Foucault, Health and Medicine*. London: Routledge, 1997.

Phleiderer, G., G. Brahier, and K. Lindpaintner (eds.). *Genethics and Religion*. Basel: Krager, 2010.

Plantinga, Alvin. *God, Freedom and Evil*. New York: Harper and Row, 1974.

Plantinga, Cornelius. *Not the Way It's Supposed To Be: A Breviary of Sin*. Grand Rapids: Eerdmans, 1995.

Pokorny, Petr. The Problem of Biblical Theology. *Horizons in Biblical Theology* 15, no. 1 (1993): 83–94.

Polanyi, Michael. *Personal Knowledge: Towards a Post-Critical Philosophy*. London: Routledge & Kegan Paul, 1958.

Pope John Paul II. *Evangelium Vitae*. Rome: Vatican, 1995.

Popper, Karl R. *Conjectures and Refutations: The Growth of Scientific Knowledge*, 4th edn. London: Routledge & Kegan Paul, 1972.

Preece, Gordon. Rethinking Singer on Life and Death. In *Rethinking Peter Singer: A Christian Critique*, edited by Gordon Preece, 122–176. Downers Grove: IVP, 2002.

Rachels, James. Active and Passive Euthanasia. In *Killing and Letting Die*, edited by Bonnie Steinbock, 63–68. Englewood Cliffs: Prentice Hall, 1980.

Radcliffe Richards, Janet. *The Ethics of Transplants: Why Careless Thought Costs Lives*. Oxford: Oxford University Press, 2012.

Räisänen, Heikki. *Beyond New Testament Theology: A Story and a Programme*. London: SCM, 1990.

Ramsey, Paul. *Ethics at the Edges of Life: Medical and Legal Intersections*. New Haven: Yale University Press, 1978.

Rickles, Dean. Public Health. In *Philosophy of Medicine*, edited by Fred Gifford, 523–572. Amsterdam: Elsevier, 2011.

Rid, Annette, and Ezekiel J. Emanuel. Ethical Considerations of Experimental Interventions in the Ebola Outbreak. *The Lancet* (2014). Published electronically 21 August 2014. http://linkinghub.elsevier.com/retrieve/pii/S0140673614613155.

Rusthoven, James. *Covenantal Biomedical Ethics for Contemporary Medicine: An Alternative to Principles-Based Ethics*. Eugene, OR: Pickwick, 2014.

Ryan, Maura. Justice and Genetics: Whose Holy Grail?. In *On Moral Medicine: Theological Perspectives in Medical Ethics*, edited by M. Therese Lysaught, Joseph J. Kotva, Jr, Stephen E. Lammers, and Allen Verhey, 973–981. Grand Rapids: Eerdmans, 2012.

Sackett, David L., William M. C. Rosenberg, J. A. Muir Gray, R. Brian Haynes, and W. Scott Richardson. Evidence-Based Medicine: What It Is and What It Isn't. *British Medical Journal* 312 (1996): 71–72.

Sadegh-Zadeh, Kazem. The Logic of Diagnosis. In *Philosophy of Medicine*, edited by Fred Gifford, 357–424. Amsterdam: Elsevier, 2011.

Sansom, Dennis. Why Do We Want to Be Healthy? Medicine, Autonomous Individualism, and the Community of Faith. *Christian Scholar's Review* 23 (1994): 300–306.

Schreiner, Thomas R. *The King in His Beauty: A Biblical Theology of the Old and New Testaments*. Grand Rapids: Baker, 2013.

Shuman, Joel, and Brian Volck. *Reclaiming the Body: Christians and the Faithful Use of Modern Medicine*. Grand Rapids: Brazos, 2006.

Sider, Ronald J. *Completely Pro-Life: Building a Consistent Stance*. Downers Grove, IL: Inter-Varsity Press, 1987.

Singer, Peter. *Practical Ethics*, 2nd edn. Cambridge: Cambridge University Press, 1993.

Singer, Peter. *Practical Ethics*. 3rd edn. Cambridge: Cambridge University Press, 2009.

Singer, Peter. *Rethinking Life and Death*. Melbourne: Text, 1994.

Sloane, Andrew. *At Home in a Strange Land: Using the Old Testament in Christian Ethics*. Peabody/Grand Rapids: Hendrickson/Baker, 2008.

Sloane, Andrew. Christianity and the Transformation of Medicine. Chapter 6 in *Christianity and the Disciplines: The Transformation of the University*, edited by Oliver D. Crisp, Gavin D'Costa, Mervyn Davies, and Peter Hampson, 85–99. London: T&T Clark, 2012.

Sloane, Andrew. Justice and the Atonement in the Book of Isaiah. *Trinity Journal* 34NS, no. 1 (2013): 3–16.

Sloane, Andrew. Justifying Advocacy: A Biblical and Theological Rationale for Speaking the Truth to Power on Behalf of the Vulnerable. *Evangelical Review of Theology* 36, no. 2 (2012): 76–86.

Sloane, Andrew. Love and Justice in International Frame. *Case* 22 (2010): 14–19.

Sloane, Andrew. The Old Testament and Christian Social Engagement. In *Another Way to Love: Christian Social Reform and Global Poverty*, edited by Tim Costello and Rod Yule, 57–72. Brunswick East: Acorn, 2009.

Sloane, Andrew. *On Being a Christian in the Academy: Nicholas Wolterstorff and the Practice of Christian Scholarship*. Carlisle: Paternoster, 2003.

Sloane, Andrew. Painful Justice: An Ethical Perspective on the Allocation of Trauma Services in Australia. *The Australian and New Zealand Journal of Surgery* 68, no. 11 (1998): 760–763.

Smith, James K. A. *Desiring the Kingdom: Worship, Worldview, and Cultural Formation*. Grand Rapids: Eerdmans, 2009.

Stark, Rodney. *The Rise of Christianity*. New York: HarperCollins, 1996.

Svenaeus, Frederik. *The Hermeneutics of Medicine and the Phenomenology of Health: Steps Towards a Philosophy of Medical Practice*. Dordrecht: Kluwer, 2010.

Tanenbaum, Sandra J. Knowing and Acting in Medical Practice: The Epistemological Politics of Outcomes Research. In *Meaning and Medicine: A Reader in the Philosophy of Health Care*, edited by J. L. Nelson and H. L. Nelson, 61–72. New York: Routledge, 1999.

Tonti-Filippini, Nicholas. Religious and Secular Death: A Parting of the Ways. *Bioethics* 26, no. 8 (2012): 410–421.

Tooley, Michael. An Irrelevant Consideration: Killing Versus Letting Die. In *Killing and Letting Die*, edited by Bonnie Steinbock, 56–62. Englewood Cliffs: Prentice Hall, 1980.

Toombs, Kay S. Chronic Illness and the Goals of Medicine. *Second Opinion* 21, no. 1 (1995): 11–19.

Uustal, Diann B. The Ethic and Spirit of Care. In *Cutting-Edge Bioethics: A Christian Exploration of Technologies and Trends*, edited by John F. Kilner, C. Christopher Hook, and Diann B. Uustal, 142–156. Grand Rapids: Eerdmans, 2002.

Veatch, Robert M. How Age Should Matter: Justice as the Basis for Limiting Care to the Elderly. In *Bioethics: An Anthology*, edited by Helga Kuhse and Peter Singer, 437–447. Oxford: Blackwell, 2006.

Verhey, Allen. Can Calvin Save Medicine? A Response to Jeff Bishop. *Christian Bioethics* 20, no. 1 (2014): 23–42.

Verhey, Allen. The Doctor's Oath – and a Christian Swearing It. In *On Moral Medicine: Theological Perspectives in Medical Ethics*, edited by M. Therese Lysaught, Joseph J. Kotva, Jr, Stephen E. Lammers, and Allen Verhey, 224–233. Grand Rapids: Eerdmans, 2012.

Verhey, Allen. *Reading the Bible in the Strange World of Medicine*. Grand Rapids: Eerdmans, 2003.

Vigen, Aana. Listening to Women of Color with Breast Cancer: Theological and Ethical Insights for US Healthcare; and 'Keeping It Real' while Staying Out of the 'Loony Bin': Social Ethics for Healthcare Systems. In *On Moral Medicine: Theological Perspectives in Medical Ethics*, edited by M. Therese Lysaught, Joseph J. Kotva, Jr, Stephen E. Lammers, and Allen Verhey, 165–184. Grand Rapids: Eerdmans, 2012.

Wartofsky, Marx. Clinical Judgment, Expert Programs, and Cognitive Style: A Counter-Essay in the Logic of Diagnosis. In *Meaning and Medicine: A Reader in the Philosophy of Health Care*, edited by J. L. Nelson and H. L. Nelson, 73–79. New York: Routledge, 1999.

Wells, Samuel. *Improvisation: The Drama of Christian Ethics*. Grand Rapids: Brazos, 2004.

Wells, Samuel. *Learning to Dream Again: Rediscovering the Heart of God*. Grand Rapids: Eerdmans, 2013.

Wolterstorff, Nicholas. Are Concept-Users World-Makers?. *Philosophical Perspectives* 1 (1987): 233–267.

Wolterstorff, Nicholas. Can Belief in God Be Rational If It Has No Foundations?. In *Faith and Rationality: Reason and Belief in God*, edited by Alvin Plantinga and Nicholas Wolterstorff, 135–186. Notre Dame: University of Notre Dame Press, 1983.

Wolterstorff, Nicholas. *Divine Discourse: Philosophical Reflections on the Claim That God Speaks*. Cambridge: Cambridge University Press, 1995.

Wolterstorff, Nicholas. Is It Possible and Desirable for Theologians to Recover from Kant? *Modern Theology* 14, no. 1 (1998): 1–18.

Wolterstorff, Nicholas. *Justice in Love*. Grand Rapids: Eerdmans, 2011.

Wolterstorff, Nicholas. *Justice: Rights and Wrongs*. Princeton: Princeton University Press, 2008.

Wolterstorff, Nicholas. The Migration of the Theistic Arguments: From Natural Theology to Evidentialist Apologetics. In *Rationality, Religious Belief, and Moral Commitment*, 38–81. Ithaca: Cornell University Press, 1986.

Wolterstorff, Nicholas. On Christian Learning. In *Stained Glass: Worldviews and Social Sciences*, edited by Paul A. Marshall, Sander Griffioen, and Richard J. Mouw, 56–80. Lanham, MD: University Press of America, 1989.

Wolterstorff, Nicholas. *Reason within the Bounds of Religion*, 2nd edn. Grand Rapids: Eerdmans, 1984.

Wolterstorff, Nicholas. *Until Justice and Peace Embrace*. Grand Rapids: Eerdmans, 1983.

Working Group. Some Issues and the Future of Theological Reflection: Reports of the Working Groups. In *Religion and Medical Ethics: Looking Back, Looking Forward*, edited by Allen Verhey, 130–141. Grand Rapids: Eerdmans, 1996.

World Health Organization. Basic Documents. Geneva, 2009.

Wright, Christopher J. H. *The Mission of God: Unlocking the Bible's Grand Narrative*. Nottingham: IVP, 2006.

Wright, Christopher J. H. *Old Testament Ethics for the People of God*. Leicester: IVP, 2004.

Wright, Tom. *Surprised by Hope*. London: SPCK, 2007.

Wyatt, John. *Matters of Life and Death: Human Dilemmas in the Light of the Christian Faith*. Nottingham: IVP, 2009.

Index